Lead, Inspire, Thrive

Fred Sanfilippo • Claire Pomeroy
David N. Bailey

Lead, Inspire, Thrive

A Handbook for Medical School Department Chairs (And Other Leaders)

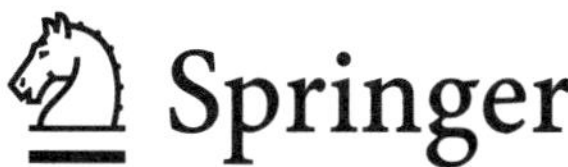

Fred Sanfilippo
Emory University
Atlanta, GA, USA

Claire Pomeroy
Lasker Foundation
New York, NY, USA

David N. Bailey
University of California San Diego
La Jolla, CA, USA

ISBN 978-3-031-41179-3   ISBN 978-3-031-41177-9   (eBook)
https://doi.org/10.1007/978-3-031-41177-9

This Springer imprint is published by the registered company Springer Nature Switzerland AG
The registered company address is: Gewerbestrasse 11, 6330 Cham, Switzerland

Paper in this product is recyclable.

The authors dedicate this book to the many past and present mentors, teachers, and advisors who have inspired us, served as role models, and guided us throughout our careers.

Fred Sanfilippo, Claire Pomeroy, and David N. Bailey

Foreword

Today is a time of unprecedented opportunity for leaders of academic health systems to promote health and improve the lives of people in communities we serve. Yet, this time is also fraught with formidable social, economic, and professional challenges. At this dynamic moment, we especially depend on medical school department chairs to stand in the spotlight and artfully conduct the orchestra of missions and constituencies that create value not only in their individual departments, but also for the academic health systems they help to lead. While there are no organizations better positioned to capitalize on the full promise of this moment than academic health systems, it is often our department chairs, with the proper preparation, who are most suited to and most heavily relied on to lead in times of opportunity and of crisis.

Medical school department chairs are key leaders and a powerful force at academic health systems across the country, who bring together the missions of health care, research, education, and community engagement in their specialties. In addition to the issues confronting the many new department chairs appointed every year, experienced chairs face the challenges of a constantly changing environment. All these department leaders have an ongoing need for answers to questions they face every day. Although the advice in these pages is targeted to new, current, and aspiring medical school department chairs, the information in this book can also be helpful to academic health system leaders of other schools, clinical services, centers, institutes, and programs.

For many chairs, the constantly evolving issues and opportunities in leading a medical school department are exciting and gratifying, but also intimidating and stressful. In addition to advancing their own careers, department chairs also must balance priorities to advance the performance of their department, the achievements of their faculty, staff, students and trainees, and the missions of their institution. This book shares extensive insights compiled by three authors who themselves have collectively served as medical school department chairs, deans, vice chancellors, and chief executive officers of academic health systems. Together, they aspire to uncover the "hidden curriculum" for department chairs to be successful in meeting the complex and sometimes conflicting expectations their faculty and their institutions have of them.

While there have been other books written for medical school department chairs, this work is novel because it poses and succinctly addresses a very wide range of questions asked by chairs and other academic health system leaders, and alerts them to issues they may not have previously considered. The Q&A format used in this book, coupled with the detailed and logical order of topics covered, provides a quick and easy way for readers to access the advice they are looking for. In addition to providing answers to the many questions addressed, the book includes a wealth of up-to-date specific references for each topic as well as a list of general references in the appendix. To facilitate use, each on-line chapter begins with an abstract summary and all the major points of each chapter are nicely summarized in the Appendix, along with a useful glossary of terms. The book provides an extensive index and is well organized to serve as a "ready reference" handbook for quick answers, as well as a comprehensive textbook on how to lead a department in an academic health system.

As a former department chair, medical school dean, university provost and chancellor, and health system chief executive officer, I find this book to be groundbreaking. It deftly captures the varied terrain of situations department chairs must be prepared to navigate. It articulately provides relevant baseline knowledge and very pertinent information for addressing a range of diverse issues. And it compellingly shares lessons that will assist chairs to effectively lead, enthusiastically inspire, and personally and professionally thrive. This is a highly valuable book that department chairs, and other leaders, will want to have in their hands as a daily-go-to reference for insight, solutions, and guidance. I am confident it will serve them well in advancing excellence and impact during this transformative time today and in the years ahead.

Duke University   A. Eugene Washington
Durham, NC, USA
September 2023

Preface

The pace of change in academic medicine is unprecedented. Medical school leaders face challenges and opportunities in all aspects of their organizations' missions of health care, research, education, and public service. Rapid change is occurring with new models of health care delivery, complex reimbursement, and health disparities; cutting-edge research technologies and approaches; innovative pedagogy and changing learning styles; and increasingly complex community needs. Furthermore, social issues such as pandemics, racial justice, climate change, and the growing use of social media and artificial intelligence (AI) tools are having considerable impact on the activity of our medical schools and the people who work there. The rapidly evolving world of academic medicine requires skilled leaders who can effectively guide today and who will prepare their faculty, staff, trainees, and students to thrive in a future that is uncertain but filled with exciting opportunities.

Medical school departments are significantly different in nature and complexity than those outside the medical school. The greater complexity is a challenge for department chairs because they must provide leadership in multiple mission areas, which serve a wide array of constituents (e.g., faculty, staff, students, researchers, educators, clinicians, patients, university, community) and have different measures of success. In addition, these missions sometimes are in direct conflict for resources across the priorities of the academic health center (AHC) or academic medical center (AMC) and its component organizations (e.g., academic units versus health care delivery systems).

Over the years, there have been numerous books offering excellent advice to academic department chairs. However, most were published more than 10 years ago when research, education, and service were much different in their organization, culture, operations, and financing. In addition, these previous publications mostly focused on advice to chairs of non-medical school departments. An exception is the Association of American Medical Colleges (AAMC) "Successful Medical School Department Chair" series. Originally published 20 years ago (2003) by Biebuyck in three modules, the series covered a variety of topics pertinent to medical school chairs at that time. Subsequently (2016, 2017, 2020) the AAMC published three new modules, each of which focused on one specific theme (leading, recruiting, and thriving, respectively). Also, *The Chronicle of Higher Education* recently prepared a compendium of its essays for department chairs (A Toolbox for Department Chairs, October 2022). All of these other works are listed in Appendix A.

Having served as medical school department chairs, program and center directors, medical school deans, and AHC/AMC chief executives, we have seen firsthand the increasing difficulty and complexity of these roles, and the need for more contemporary and comprehensive advice to help medical school department chairs navigate the many issues and opportunities they face. Two of us (FS and DNB) also have led a group of former medical school department chairs whose primary mission is to mentor and advise department leaders as well as those aspiring to become leaders, resulting in several recent papers providing advice and addressing questions raised.

While serving as a medical school department chair is challenging on many levels, it is one of the most important roles in AHCs and AMCs, and can be an extremely rewarding leadership position. As we have learned during our own careers and from observing others, timely advice and mentorship are keys to success. Therefore, we wish to share these insights by articulating and answering the most common questions posed by medical school department chairs and other leaders over their careers. We also include summaries in Appendix D that highlight key points in each chapter and section for a quick and handy reference.

This book aims to provide easily accessible advice to new, experienced, and aspiring medical school chairs, regardless of the particular organizational structure in which they function, as well as AHC and AMC leaders in other schools, centers, programs, research institutes, and clinical services. Whether it is used to answer specific questions or read in its entirety, this book is designed as a guide for those who are leaders in their organization to help them inspire stakeholders and thrive personally and professionally in these key roles.

Atlanta, GA, USA
New York, NY, USA
La Jolla, CA, USA Fred Sanfilippo
Claire Pomeroy
David N. Bailey

Acknowledgments

As a reflection of our personal experience and benefit from the many teachers, mentors, and coaches who have provided advice and assistance we have many individuals to recognize and thank for the lessons learned that we have used in this book.

Fred Sanfilippo is grateful to the teachers who had lasting impact from his early years of schooling, especially for the advice and encouragement of Peter Backus at Molloy High School, J. Heinrich Matthaei for the extraordinary opportunity, support, and training he provided at the Max Plank Institute for Experimental Medicine, and Alan Heeger and Tony Garito for providing career counseling and mentorship during his Master's research at Penn about how physics and medical interdisciplinary research could enhance innovation and create opportunities. Many teachers, mentors, and role models provided important career lessons at Duke, especially Thomas D. Kinney, who showed how deans should focus their attention on students, the importance of DEI in medical education, and for the many opportunities he created; William Anlyan, for showing how to lead and delegate to teams (and be a good tennis partner), Bernard Amos for showing how to think out of the box for highest impact, David Scott for how to be a mensch, David Sabiston for the resources he provided to keep him at Duke and how to always strive for excellence, and Robert Jennings for how to be gracious and supportive of the institution even when priorities change. Several mentors at Hopkins provided important lessons in leadership, especially Cathy DeAngelis for how to value diversity and mentor faculty, Mike Johns for how to support leaders and provide them opportunities, and John Cameron for how to get things done. He also thanks leaders and colleagues at Ohio State, especially Brit Kirwan for showing how best to recruit and retain talent, Pete Geier for how to bring competing departments and people together, Tony Rucci for how to value faculty and staff behavior relative to their achievements, Frank LaFasto for how to build and support teams, Jay Barney for how organizational structure and culture can transform performance, Sue Jablonski for how to communicate effectively, and Gail Marsh for how to develop effective strategies and tactics. He also thanks Bob Walter for showing how important it is to balance work and personal life activities with family and friends, Bernie Marcus for how to raise and use funds effectively, and Len Schlesinger for showing how to think strategically, improve performance, and focus on priorities. Most importantly, he is forever grateful to his wife Janet, who has been his major source of strength and support for over 50 years.

Claire Pomeroy is grateful for the many mentors, colleagues, and students who have made her career in medicine so gratifying and inspiring. She thanks Jim Mitchell for the opportunity to be part of the team treating and researching eating disorders at the University of Minnesota (U-Minn); Colin Jordan and Greg Filice for their mentorship during her training in infectious disease at U-Minn; and Randy Petzel for his support of establishing the first HIV Clinic at the Minneapolis VA. She is indebted to Dick Glassock and Emery Wilson for the numerous opportunities provided to her for career development at the University of Kentucky, including pursuing an MBA degree. She thanks Joe Silva for recruiting her to the University of California, Davis, and encouraging her career development and selection as his successor as dean. Over the past 10 years, she has been fortunate to work with dedicated board chairs at the Albert and Mary Lasker Foundation—Al Sommer, Mike Overlock, and Tony Evnin and an amazing array of leaders on the board of directors. She is grateful to her colleagues on corporate boards who welcomed and guided her in a new career direction. Her professional journey has been exciting and continues to lead to new and sometimes unexpected learning, in large part due to the mentors, mentees, and colleagues with whom she has the privilege of interacting. She thanks her husband, William Preston Robertson, for his steadfast support and encouragement.

David Bailey is grateful for the mentorship of David Seligson, founding chair of the Department of Laboratory Medicine at Yale University, in whose laboratories he worked from his first days as a medical student, and who sparked a desire to pursue an academic career. He is also immensely thankful for the inspiration provided by Peter Jatlow, the second chair of that department, who nurtured his research interests and taught him how to prepare his first manuscripts for publication while a medical student and subsequently a resident and fellow. The seemingly countless manuscript revisions requested by Peter, while frustrating (without word processing in those days!), taught him how to write and edit successfully. He also is grateful to Alfred Zettner, founding Head of the Division of Laboratory Medicine, for recruiting him to the University of California San Diego (UC San Diego), where he found unlimited opportunities for personal growth as an academician. He particularly acknowledges Peter Lampert, third chair of the Department of Pathology at UC San Diego, who provided him with his initial leadership opportunities as director of clinical laboratories, division head, and executive vice chair of the department. Following Peter's untimely death, he succeeded him as department chair, utilizing the many lessons learned from him while holding the department together and leading it forward during particularly challenging times. Finally, he thanks Edward Holmes, former UC San Diego Vice Chancellor and medical school dean, who taught him valuable lessons in how to be a successful dean and vice chancellor.

The authors appreciate and acknowledge the many colleagues who helped advise us on the content, preparation, and publication of this book including Ralph Hruban, Steven Klasko, Priscilla Markwood, Swetha Rajagopalan, Janet Sanfilippo, Guido Silvestri, and Len Schlesinger. We also are grateful for the guidance and assistance provided to us by the extraordinary staff at Springer Nature in the publication of this book, with particular thanks to Jessica Chio (Associate Editor), Richard Lansing (Editorial Director), Rekha Muthusamy (Project Coordinator), and Shaik Safha (Project Manager).

Finally, we acknowledge the stimulation, collaboration, and satisfaction we have provided to each other in the planning and writing of this book. We have learned much from each other.

Fred Sanfilippo
Claire Pomeroy
David N. Bailey

Contents

1 Introduction 1
  References 3

Part I Getting Started

2 Setting Initial Goals 7
  Starting Out 7
    "What Is the Scope of My Authority and Responsibilities
    as Chair?" 7
    "What Should My "Chair Package" Include?" 8
    "What Are the Key Things to Remember as a New Department
    Chair?" 9
    "How Do I Determine What I Need to Know to Fulfill My New
    Role?" 9
    "What Goals Should I Set for My First 100 Days,
    Especially If Moving to a New Institution?" 9
  Your Initial Message: First Impressions Are Lasting 10
    "Upon Being Appointed Chair, How and
    What Should I Communicate to Members of My Department
    and Institutional Leaders?" 10
    "How Should I Communicate Expectations of the Institution
    to My Department?" 11
  Getting the Faculty and Staff Involved 12
    "How Can I Best Engage My Faculty and Staff in Setting Goals
    During My First 100 Days?" 12
  Getting External Help in Setting Goals 12
    "Whom Should I Involve from Outside the Department to Help
    Set Initial Goals?" 12
  References 13

3   Expectations.   15
      Measuring Your Success   15
          "How Do I Best Determine the Institutional Measures of Success
          for Me and My Department?".   15
          "How Do I Best Determine the Departmental Measures of Success
          for Me and the Department?"   16
          "How Should I Determine Personal Measures of Success for Me
          and the Department?"   16
      Serving as an Interim Chair   16
          "Should I Consider Serving as an Interim Chair?".   16
          "How Might Expectations Be Affected If I'm Serving as an
          Interim Versus a Permanent Chair?".   17
          "Will Expectations About My Role as an Interim Chair Hurt
          or Improve My Chances of Becoming Permanent Leader?"   17
      "Internal" Versus "External" Recruitment   18
          "How Might Expectations Be Affected If I Was an
          Internal Candidate for the Chair Versus an External Candidate?" . . .   18
      Prior Leadership Experience.   18
          "How Might Expectations Be Affected If I've Previously
          Served as a Chair?".   18
      Surprises   19
          "What Should I Watch Out for After Assuming My Role as New
          Chair?"   19
      References.   20

4   Dealing with Your Predecessor   21
      Developing a Relationship   21
          "How Should I Interact with a Former Chair?"   21
      Advice and Assistance   22
          "When Should I Ask the Former Chair for Help and Advice?"   22
      Dealing with Interference   23
          "How Should I Deal with Problems Created
          by My Predecessor?"   23
      References.   23

Part II   Interpersonal Interactions, Culture, and Behavior

5   Communication.   27
      Enhancing Your Communication Skills   27
          "How Can I Improve My Speaking Skills?".   27
          "How Can I Improve My Writing Skills?"   28
          "How and When Should I Use Different Types
          of Communication?".   29
          "How Much Should I Read into Body Language?"   29

Transparency and Establishing Trust   30
   "How Can I Best Maintain Communication to Establish Trust
   and Confidence?"   30
   "How Do I Promote Feedback and Constructive Advice
   from My Department and Institutional Leaders?"   31
   "How Should I Deal with Gossip and Rumors About
   Departmental and Institutional Leaders and Their Decisions?"   32
   "How Should I Handle Freedom of Speech and Academic
   Freedom Issues That May Come Up?"   32
Accommodating Institutional Priorities and Reforms   33
   "How Do I Communicate Institutional Priorities and Decisions
   to My Faculty and Staff, Especially When I Personally Disagree
   with Them?"   33
   "How Do I Advocate for My Department During Institutional
   Reallocation of Resources, Curriculum Changes, Etc.?"   34
   "How Do I Best Prepare My Faculty for a Significant Change
   in the Department, School, University, or AHC/AMC?"   34
References   34

6   Organizational Culture   35
Understanding Culture Types and Styles   35
   "What Do I Need to Know About Organizational Culture?"   35
   "What Are the Different Culture Types and Styles
   of Which I Should Be Aware?"   35
Evaluating Your Organizational Culture(s)   36
   "How Can I Evaluate the Culture of My Department?"   36
   "How Do I Determine If the Culture in My Department
   Needs to Change?"   37
Driving Culture Change   37
   "How Can I Improve the Culture of My Department?"   37
Promoting Teamwork   38
   "How Can I Develop and Improve Teamwork
   in My Department?"   38
References   38

7   Diversity, Equity, and Inclusion   41
Highlighting the Importance of Diversity, Equity,
and Inclusion (DEI)   41
   "How Can I Highlight the Importance of DEI
   for My Department?"   41
DEI Education and Training   42
   "What Are the Best Ways to Provide Training About DEI
   in My Department?"   42
Enhancing and Promoting DEI   43
   "How Do I Promote and Enhance DEI in My Department?"   43

"How Do I Ensure That Departmental Practices Support
Recruitment of Diverse Candidates?"   44
"What Are Best Practices for Enhancing an Inclusive
and Equitable Culture in My Department?"   44
"How Can Career Development Programs Help Advance DEI
in My Department?"   45
"How Do I Avoid Exacting 'Gender or Minority Taxes'?"   45
Measuring Success   46
"How Should I Monitor DEI in My Department?"   46
References   46

8   Building Collaborations and Collegiality   49
The Value Added   49
"What Are the Benefits of Promoting Faculty Collaboration
and Collegiality?"   49
Research and Clinical Faculty Relationships   50
"How Can I Encourage Collaboration Between Research
and Clinical Faculty?"   50
Stimulating Collaboration   51
"What Are Appropriate Incentives to Stimulate Collaboration?"   51
Promoting Collegiality   51
"How Should I Promote Collegiality?"   51
References   52

9   Promoting Work-Life Balance   53
Developing a Successful Departmental Work-Life Balance   53
"How Can I Promote a Successful Work-Life Balance
for Members of My Department?"   53
Work Time   54
"How Can I Help Members of My Department Better Manage
Their Administrative Work Time?"   54
"How Can I Help Members of My Department Better Manage
Their Professional Work Time?"   55
Personal Time   55
"How Can I Help Members of My Department Better Utilize
and Appreciate the Importance of Personal Time?"   55
References   56

10   Negotiation   57
When to Negotiate   57
"When Should I Negotiate Rather Than Just Agree
with a Proposal or Counter-Proposal?"   57
"When Should I Start a New Negotiation in Response
to a Proposal?"   57

How to Negotiate   58
   "How Should I Negotiate for Departmental Resources
   Such as Budget, Space, Personnel, Etc.?"   58
   "How Should I Negotiate When Dealing with Faculty
   and Staff Requests for Resources, Promotion, Etc.?"   58
   "How Should I Negotiate for Personal Issues Such as Salary,
   Space, Staff Support, Etc.?"   59
  "Do's and Don'ts"   59
  References   59

Part III   Operational Issues

11   Organizing the Department   63
  Leadership Positions   63
   "What Leadership Positions Should I Keep, Change,
   and Create?"   63
  Building Your Team   64
   "Should I Create a Departmental Leadership Team
   (e.g., 'Executive Committee'), and, If So, What Should Be
   Its Composition and Its Role?"   64
   "How Should I Delegate Authority to My Faculty
   and Administrative Leaders?"   65
   "How Should I Interact with My Faculty and Administrative
   Leaders?"   66
  Divisions and Sections   67
   "What Are Successful Departmental Organizational Models?"   67
   "Should I Restructure the Department?"   68
  Operations and Administration   68
   "How Should I Organize Administrative Staff to Best Support
   the Activities of the Department?"   68
   "How Do I Align Departmental Administrators and Staff
   Who Report to Different Parent Organizations
   (e.g., Hospital, University Campus)?"   69
  Meetings and Events   69
   "How Should I Schedule and Utilize Departmental Meetings?"   69
   "What Events Should I Consider Scheduling for the Department?" .   70
   "What Meetings Should I Consider Attending Personally?"   71
   "How Should I Participate in Meetings?"   71
  References   71

12   Strategic Planning   73
  Evaluating Your Departmental Strategic Plan   73
   "What Is the Best Approach for Reviewing My Department's
   Current Strategic Plan?"   73
   "What If I Think the Current Departmental Plan Needs to Be
   Revised or Completely Redone?"   74

Refreshing an Existing Strategic Plan.   74
"What If I Am Expected to Implement the Current Departmental
Plan But Believe That It Is Inadequate?"   74
Developing a New Strategic Plan   75
"When Should I Launch a New Departmental Strategic Planning
Process?".   75
"What If I Am Expected to Lead the Development
and Implementation of a New Plan But Find Substantial
Departmental Resistance?".   76
"How Should I Develop and Implement a New Strategic Plan?". . . .   76
Managing Change.   77
"What Should I Know About Managing Change?"   77
"How Can I Manage the Changes Needed in My Department?"   78
References.   79

13   **Resources**   81
Resource Management   81
"How Should I Prioritize Allocation of My Limited Departmental
Resources (People, Space, Funding) to Meet the Substantial
Demands?"   81
People   82
"With So Many Departmental Needs and Opportunities,
How Should I Prioritize Recruitment and Retention of Faculty
and Staff?".   82
"When Should I Consider Joint Recruitment or Retention
of Faculty or Staff with Another Department or Center?"   82
"How Should I Allocate Resources to Support Faculty?"   83
Space.   84
"Is the Current Space Allocation in My Department Appropriate?" .   84
"How Do I Take Space Away from a Faculty Member?"   84
"How Best to Relocate Faculty and Staff into New Space?"   85
Funding.   85
"What Should I Know About Departmental and Institutional
Funds Flow?"   85
References.   86

14   **Budgets and Finance**.   87
Assessing Departmental Finances.   87
"What Should I Know About My Departmental Finances?"   87
"What Should I Know About My Institutional Finances?"   87
"What Should My Department Know About Departmental
Finances?".   88
"What Institutional Policies Can Affect My Departmental
Finances?".   88
Sources and Uses   89
"How Should I Prioritize Spending?".   89
"How Can I Be Flexible with Expenses?"   90

Developing a Budget. 91
"What Is the Best Budget Process for My Department?". 91
"What Assumptions Should I Make When Budgeting?" 91
Margins and Deficits. 92
"How Should I Use Unexpected Financial Margins?" 92
"How Should I Deal with an Unexpected Financial Deficit?" 92
References. 93

15 Balancing the Missions. 95
The Balancing Act. 95
"How Do I Successfully Balance the Research, Clinical,
Education, and Public Service Missions of the Department?" 95
Your Involvement in Each Mission. 96
"To What Extent Should I as Leader Be Directly Engaged
in Clinical Service, Research, and Teaching, Given
My Administrative Duties and Responsibilities?" 96
Alignment of Missions 96
"How Can I Ensure That the Missions of My Department
Are Properly Aligned?". 96
References. 97

16 Crisis Management. 99
General 99
"How Should I Deal with a Significant and Unexpected Crisis
in My Department?" 99
Financial 100
"What Should I Do If My Department Has a Significant
and Unexpected Budget Problem?" 100
Environmental. 100
"How Should I Prioritize Activities During an Environmental
Crisis?" 100
Personal. 101
"How Should I Prioritize My Activities During a Personal
Crisis?" 101
Opportunities to Learn from Crises 101
"What Lessons Can Be Learned from Crises?" 101
References. 102

Part IV Faculty Issues

17 Faculty Recruitment and Retention 105
Recruiting New Faculty 105
"When and How Should I Start a Search for a New Faculty
Member?". 105
"Should I Use a Search Firm?". 107
"What Best Practices Are Recommended for Appointing Search
Committees?" 107

"What Start-Up Resources Should I Consider for New Faculty?"... 108
"What Are Effective Ways to Interact with Candidates?" 108
"What Should I Consider When Onboarding New Faculty
Recruits?" 109
Retaining Current Talent.. 110
"What Are Effective Strategies for Retaining Faculty
Who Consider Leaving Your Department?" 110
Closing the Deal 110
"What Are Some of the Issues I Should Consider to Be
Successful in Faculty Recruitment and Retention?".............. 110
"Should I Make a Special Deal to Recruit or Retain a Special
or Extraordinary Individual?"................................. 111
Appointments, Promotions, and Tenure 111
"What Should I Know About the Faculty Appointments,
Promotions, and Tenure (APT) Process at My Institution?" 111
"What Are Some Issues That Can Arise with Faculty
Appointments?" 112
"What Are Some Issues That Can Arise with Faculty Promotions
and Tenure?".. 113
"What About Clinical Faculty Who Are Hospital Employees?" 113
"What About Emeriti Faculty and Volunteer Faculty?" 114
References... 115

18   Faculty Career Development and Wellness 117
Resources for Career Development 117
"Where Can I Find Programs That Can Help the Career
Development of My Faculty?" 117
Implementing Career Development Programs 118
"How Can I Set Up an Effective Department-Wide Career
Development Program?"...................................... 118
Expanding Faculty Productivity 118
"How Can I Help Faculty Increase Their Productivity?" 118
"How Do I Determine the Proper Use of Virtual and Remote
Work for Faculty?" 119
Enhancing Wellness 120
"What Are Best Practices in Implementing a Faculty Wellness
Program?"... 120
Reviewing Performance 121
"What Are Best Practices in Conducting Faculty Reviews?"....... 121
"What Are Problems That Can Occur with Reviews,
and How Should I Deal with Them?"........................... 122
References... 122

19 Faculty Compensation Plans 125
   Characteristics.. 125
      "How Do I Ensure That Our Departmental Compensation
      Plan Is Equitable for Faculty Based on Their Activities
      and Performance?" 125
   Incentives and Bonuses...................................... 126
      "What Activities Should I Include in an Incentive Plan?" 126
   Review Process... 127
      "How Should I Evaluate Performance and Productivity
      to Determine Appropriate Compensation?" 127
      "How Should I Deal with Compensation for Clinical Faculty
      Who Want to Maintain Their High Salary but Reduce Their
      Clinical Load to Get a Grant or Pursue More Academic
      Activities?" 128
      "How Should I Deal with Compensation for a Research
      Faculty Member Who Receives or Loses a Significant Grant?"..... 128
      "How Should I Deal with Compensation for a Faculty
      Member Who Is No Longer Productive?" 128
   References.. 129

20 Dealing with Difficult Faculty 131
   Considerations.. 131
      "What Factors Should I Consider When Dealing with a
      Difficult Faculty Member?" 131
   Evaluation... 132
      "How Should I Evaluate a Problem Individual?" 132
   Resolution... 132
      "How Should I Resolve Issues with Difficult Faculty?"........... 132
   Mistakes 133
      "What Are Some of the Serious Mistakes I Can Make
      in Dealing with Problem Faculty?"........................... 133
   References.. 133

Part V Student and Trainee Issues

21 Student and Trainee Recruitment............................. 137
   Attracting the Right Students and Trainees 137
      "How Do I Interest Medical Students and Other Health
      Profession Students in Doing Rotations in My Department?"...... 137
      "How Do I Attract and Recruit the Best Residents
      and Fellows to My Department?"............................ 138
      "How Do I Support Faculty to Be Competitive for Attracting MS
      and PhD Students, as well as Post-doctoral Scholars in My
      Department?" 138

Providing a High-Quality Learning Environment.   139
  "What Is My Role as Chair in Helping to Shape the Curriculum
  for Students?"   139
  "How Do I Ensure that Residents and Fellows Receive
  Effective Training in My Department?"   140
  "How Much Influence Should I Have on the Experience
  of MS and PhD Students and Post-doctoral Researchers?"   140
  "How Can I Promote Diversity and Inclusion in the Learning
  Environment for Students and Trainees in My Department?"   141
  "What Should I Do if Students or Trainees Want to Lodge
  Concerns or Complaints About Their Experience
  in My Department?"   141
  "How Can I Optimize CME Programs Offered
  by My Departmental Faculty?".   142
Providing Compensation and Benefits   142
  "How Are Salaries for Trainees Set? How Do I Ensure
  that the Pay Is Reasonable?.   142
  "What Is My Role in Overseeing the Compensation
  Received by Post-doctoral Scholars in My Department?"   143
References.   143

22 Student and Trainee Career Development and Wellness   145
Resources for Career Development   145
  "What Programming Should My Department Provide
  for Students' and Trainees' Career Development?"   145
  "How Can I Shape the Student and Trainee Experience
  in My Department in a Way That Attracts Them
  to Our Specialty or Institution upon Graduation?".   146
Enhancing Achievement   146
  "What Is My Role as Chair in the Development
  and Delivery of the Curriculum in My Department?"   146
  "What Characteristics of the Learning Environment
  Are Important for Achieving Student Success?"   146
  "How Can I Ensure That Trainees Achieve Their Full
  Potential Through the Experiences Offered in My Department?" . . .   147
Promoting Wellness   147
  "How Can the Department Enhance Wellness Among
  the Medical and Other Health Profession Students and Trainees
  in My Department?"   147
  "What Do I Do When a Student or Trainee Manifests
  a Mental Health Issue?"   148
Reviewing Performance   148
  "What Are Good Approaches for Evaluating Student
  and Trainee Performance in My Department?"   148

"How Do I Ensure That Students and Trainees Are Being
Accurately and Fairly Evaluated by the Faculty
in My Department?"   149
"What Should I Do When Suboptimal Performance
by a Student or Trainee Is Reported or Observed?"   149
References   150

23 Dealing with Difficult Students and Trainees   151
Considerations   151
"Whose Responsibility Is It to Address Student or Trainee
Problems?"   151
Evaluation   152
"What Resources Are Available for Me to Help Students/Trainees
Who Are Experiencing Difficulties in My Department?"   152
"What Is My Responsibility for Monitoring Trends in Student
and/or Trainee Performance Difficulties in My Department?"   152
Resolution   152
"What Is the Best Approach to Remedying Problems Identified
in Student and Trainee Performance?"   152
"How Do I Respond to Inquiries from Another Institution
or a Potential Employer About Students/Trainees Who Have
Performed Poorly or Been Disciplined?"   153
Mistakes   153
"To Whom and How Should I Disclose Information About
Students/Trainees Who Make Clinical Errors or Violate
Research Regulations?"   153
References   154

Part VI Staff Issues

24 Staff Recruitment and Retention   157
Identifying the Right People for the Jobs   157
"Should I Keep My Predecessor's Staff?"   157
"How Do I Build My Own Team of High-Functioning Staff
for My Department?"   157
Recruiting New Staff   159
"When Should I Recruit from Inside the Institution
and When Should I Look Outside?"   159
"How Can I Enhance DEI for Staff in My Department?"   159
Retaining Current Staff   160
"What Are Tips for Keeping Talented Staff in the Department?"   160
"When Should Remote Work Be Considered for Staff Members?" ..   161
References   161

25 Staff Career Development and Wellness 163

Career Development, Succession Planning, and Training 163

"How Should I Support the Career Development of Key Staff
Members in My Department?" 163

"What About Succession Planning for Staff?" 164

Enhancing Productivity 164

"How Can I Incentivize My Team to Be a High-Performing
Group?" 164

Promoting Wellness 165

"How Can I Help Staff Thrive in My Department?" 165

Reviewing Performance 165

"What Are Best Practices for Reviewing the Performance
of Departmental Staff? 165

"Should I Delegate Performance Reviews to Others?" 166

References 166

26 Staff Compensation 167

Salaries and Benefits 167

"How Are Salaries and Benefits Set for Staff
in My Department?" 167

"What Do I Need to Consider if My Staff Are Represented
by Unions?" 167

"How Do I Deal with the Fact That Contracted Employees
(e.g., Traveling Nurses) May Be Paid Substantially More
than Staff Employees?" 168

Work Assignments 169

"How Do I Ensure That Expectations of Staff Are Fair
and Linked Appropriately to Compensation?" 169

"What Do I Do When Unionized Staff Go on Strike?" 169

Monitoring Staff Compensation Levels and Equity 169

"How Do I Ensure That Staff Compensation Is Equitable
and Competitive?" 169

"What Are My Options if Compensation Is Below Market
or Insufficient to Attract the Staff Talent I Need
in My Department?" 170

"What Are the Challenges and Best Approaches
to Having Both Staff (Nonfaculty) Physicians
and Faculty Physicians in My Department?" 170

References 171

27 Dealing with Difficult or Unproductive Staff 173

Considerations 173

"When Should I Deal with Difficult or Unproductive Staff
Personally and When Should I Involve Others?" 173

Evaluation and Resolution   174
   "What Policies Apply to Dealing with Staff Who Are Not
   Performing Well or Experiencing Personal or Interpersonal Issues?"   174
   "What Resources Are Available for Me to Help Staff
   Who Are Experiencing Difficulties in My Department?".   175
   "How Should Staff Performance Be Monitored
   in My Department?"   175
Mistakes   175
   "What Is the Best Approach to Deal with Staff Members
   Who Make Serious Mistakes in the Performance
   of Their Duties?".   175
   "How Do I Respond to Requests for Job References About
   Staff Who Have Left the Department Under Adverse
   Circumstances?"   176
References.   176

Part VII   Interactions Beyond Your Department

28   Interacting with Institutional Leaders   179
Understanding Your Institutional Leadership Teams   179
   "What Should I Know About Leadership at My Institution(s)?"   179
Working with Your Institutional Leaders   180
   "How Do I Develop a Positive Relationship with
   Those to Whom I Report?"   180
   "How Should I Bring Problems or Requests to My Bosses?"   181
Being a Team Player   181
   "How Do I Balance My Role as Department Chair with Being
   an Institutional Team Player?"   181
References.   182

29   Interdepartmental Interactions   183
Working with Peer Institutional Leaders   183
   "How Can I Build Productive Relationships
   with My Peer Institutional Leaders?"   183
Developing Joint Programs.   184
   "What Are Ways to Build Synergistic Interdepartmental
   Programs?"   184
Resources and Recognition.   186
   "How Can I Best Obtain and Use Resources
   for Interdepartmental Programs?"   186
   "How Can I Best Promote the 'Purview' of My Department
   in a Constructive Manner and Without Offending Colleagues
   in Other Departments?"   186

Dealing with Interdepartmental Conflicts.   187
"How Should I Deal with Conflicts Between My Department
and Other Departments and Centers?"   187
References.   188

30 Departmental and Institutional Alignment   189
Determining Priorities.   189
"How Should I Determine the Appropriate Priorities for My
Department?"   189
Misalignment with Institutional Mission and Vision   190
"How Should I Deal with Misalignment of My Department
Mission and Vision with Those of a Parent Institution?"   190
Building Alignment.   190
"How Can I Build Alignment Between My Department
and Institutional Leadership Regarding Mission and Vision?".   190
"How Should I Deal with Changes in Institutional Priorities
and Use of Resources?"   191
References.   191

31 Interactions with External Entities   193
Getting Institutional Approval   193
"When and How Should I Get Institutional Approval
for External Interactions?"   193
Universities   194
"How Can I Take Advantage of Potential Opportunities
for My Department with Other Universities?"   194
"What Issues Should I Consider When Interacting
with Other Universities?"   194
Hospitals and Health Systems.   195
"What Are the Major Considerations When Interacting
with Hospitals?"   195
"How Can I Take Advantage of Potential Opportunities
at Other Hospitals?"   195
"What Are Some of the Risks of Interacting with Other
Hospitals?"   195
"Are There Special Hospital Affiliations That I Should
Consider for My Department?"   196
Professional Societies   196
"How Can I Take Advantage of Working with Professional
Societies?".   196
"What Are Some of the Issues to Consider with Professional
Society Interactions?".   197
Non-Profit Organizations   198
"What Are Issues to Consider in Working with Non-Profit
Organizations?".   198

Companies.. 198
  "How Can My Department Take Advantage of Working
  with For-Profit Companies?".. 198
  "What Are Some of the Risks and Problems of Working
  with Companies?"... 199
Community Leaders... 199
  "How Can I Best Engage Productively with Community
  Leaders?".. 199
  "What Are Some of the Risks and Problems in Dealing
  with Community Leaders?"... 200
The Media.. 201
  "How Do I Best Engage with the Media?"........................... 201
  "What Are Some of the Risks and Problems in Dealing
  with the Media?".. 201
References... 202

32 Fundraising and Donor Development............................... 203
Identifying Uses... 203
  "What Activities Should I Target for Departmental Fundraising?".. 203
  "What Activities Should I Avoid for Departmental Fundraising?"... 204
Developing Donors... 204
  "How Should I Engage Potential Donors?"......................... 204
  "What Attracts Potential Donors?"................................. 205
  "What Do Potential Donors Worry About?"......................... 206
  "Whom Should I Try to Develop as Donors to My Department?"... 207
  "How Do I Deal with Conflicts Over Donors with Whom Other
  Departments or the Institution Are Engaging?".................... 207
Dealing with Foundations.. 208
  "How Do I Deal with Foundations?"................................ 208
Creating a Development Program for Your Department.............. 209
  "How Do I Build a Successful Departmental Development
  Program?"... 209
  "How Much of My Own Time Should I Allocate to
  Fundraising and Donor Development?"............................. 210
References... 210

Part VIII Personal Issues

33 Leadership Attributes.. 213
Characteristics of Successful Leaders................................. 213
  "Why Should I Want to Be a Department Chair?"................. 213
  "What Are the Behaviors, Skills, and Style of Successful
  Leaders?".. 213
  "How Do I Lead in the Rapidly Changing World of Academic
  Medicine?".. 215

Evaluation of Leadership Skills 216
  "How Do I Know If I Have the Skills of a Successful Leader?" 216
Developing and Maintaining Self-Awareness..................... 216
  "How Do I Become More Self-Aware of My Own Strengths
  and Weaknesses?".. 216
  "How Should I Deal with Mistakes?".......................... 217
Leadership Training 217
  "Where Can I Obtain Formal Leadership Training?"............. 217
Dealing with Criticism 218
  "How Should I Handle Criticism?" 218
Handling Conflicts of Interest................................. 219
  "How Should I Handle Conflicts of Interest?" 219
Maintaining Confidentiality 220
  "How Do I Know What to Keep Confidential and What I May
  Disclose?"... 220
References.. 220

34 Getting Advice and Assistance.............................. 223
Advisors and Consultants 223
  "When Should I Use an Advisor or a Consultant?" 223
  "How Do I Find the Right Advisor or Consultant to Help Me
  with a Specific Issue?" 224
Mentors... 225
  "How Should I Find and Develop a Relationship with a Mentor?" .. 225
Coaches... 225
  "When Do I Need Coaching?" 225
  "How Do I Find the Right Coach for Me?" 226
Sponsors 226
  "What Is a Sponsor and How Can I Find an Appropriate One?" 226
Family and Friends 226
  "When Should I Ask Family and Friends for Advice?" 226
References.. 227

35 Handling Reviews 229
Dealing with Personal Reviews 229
  "How Should I Approach My Annual Review?" 229
  "How Should I Respond to Personal Recommendations
  in My Department Review?" 230
  "How Should I Handle a Targeted Review of My Performance or
  Behavior?" 230
Purpose of Department Reviews................................. 231
  "What Are the Expectations of a Department Review?" 231
Preparing for a Department Review 232
  "How Do I Get Ready for a Review of My Department?"......... 232

Review "Etiquette"   233
  "What Are the 'Do's and Don'ts' for Me in the Department
  Review Process?"   233
Dealing with the Review Report.   233
  "How Should I React to the Review Report, Especially
  If It Is Not Entirely Positive?"   233
Dealing with Program and Institution Reviews   234
  "How Should I Handle Program, Accreditation, and
  Institution Reviews That Involve My Department?"   234
References.   235

36 Achieving Work-Life Balance   237
Importance of Work-Life Balance   237
  "How Can I Achieve a Successful Work-Life Balance?"   237
  "As a Department Chair, Should I Even Consider Taking
  a Sabbatical Leave?"   238
Time Management at Work.   239
  "What Are Strategies for Managing My Work Schedule?"   239
Handling Appointments   240
  "How Can I Handle All the Appointments Requested?"   240
  "How Can I Use Meeting Time More Effectively?".   240
Enhancing Resilience   241
  "How Can I Increase My Resilience to Stress?".   241
Time for Family and Friends.   241
  "How Can I Ensure That My Work Schedule Does Not
  Preclude Time with Family and Friends?"   241
Personal Time   242
  "How Can I Find Time Just to Relax and Have Fun?"   242
References.   243

37 Career Transitioning.   245
Knowing When It's Time   245
  "How Do I Know When It Is Time to Transition?"   245
  "How Long Is Too Long to Serve as a Department Leader?"   246
Considering Options.   246
  "What Transition Opportunities Should I Consider?"   246
Imposed Termination   247
  "How Best to Transition from an Imposed Termination?"   247
Succession Planning   248
  "When Should I Start My Succession Planning
  for My Department?"   248
Coping with Transition   248
  "How Do I Deal with No Longer Being the Department
  Leader?"   248
References.   249

38   Changing Positions 251
  Becoming a Candidate 251
    "How Do I Become a Candidate for an Attractive Position
    Without Damaging My Current Department?". 251
  Interviews and Visits. 252
    "How Do I Handle Interviews and Visits for Another Position
    While I'm Still Running My Department?" 252
  Evaluating the Opportunity. 253
    "How Do I Determine If Taking a New Position
    Is the Right Change to Make?". 253
  Closing the Deal 253
    "How Should I Finalize the Agreement for My New Position?" 253
  Leaving Gracefully 254
    "How Do I Make the Right Exit from My Current
    Position to Another One?" 254
  Expect Surprises 254
    "Did I Make the Right Decision in Changing Positions? 254
  References. 255

Final Thoughts. 257

**Appendix A: Other Works Offering Advice for Academic
Department Chairs**. 259

Appendix B: References for General Reading 261

Appendix C: Glossary of Terms Used 263

Appendix D: Chapter Summaries 269

Index. 315

About the Authors

Fred Sanfilippo, MD, PhD, is Director of the Emory-Georgia Tech Healthcare Innovation Program, Professor of Pathology & Laboratory Medicine, and Health Policy & Management at Emory University where he served as Executive VP for Health Affairs, CEO of the Woodruff Health Sciences Center, and Board Chair of Emory Healthcare.

From 2000 to 2007 he served Ohio State University as Senior VP and Executive Dean for Health Sciences, Medical Center CEO, Dean of the College of Medicine and Public Health, and Board Chair of Managed Health Care Systems. From 1993 to 2000, he was the Baxley Professor, Chair of Pathology and Pathologist-in-Chief at Johns Hopkins. He led the formation of the Johns Hopkins Medical Labs and the Johns Hopkins Comprehensive Transplant Center, serving as its first Research Director. From 1979 to 1993 he was a faculty member at Duke University, rising to Professor of Pathology, Experimental Surgery, and Immunology.

He received BS and MSc degrees in physics from the University of Pennsylvania, MD and PhD (immunology) from Duke University where he did his residency training with board certifications in Anatomic-Clinical Pathology and Immunopathology. Among his many honors he has received Distinguished Alumni Awards from Duke and Johns Hopkins Universities, and been elected president of seven professional organizations including the American Society of Investigative Pathology and the American Society of Transplantation.

Providing advice, mentorship, and coaching to students, trainees, faculty, staff, deans, and AHC/AMC leaders has been a major priority for Dr. Sanfilippo, who also has consulted for scores of foundations, NGOs, companies, and government agencies.

Claire Pomeroy, MD, MBA, is president and CEO of the Albert and Mary Lasker Foundation since 2013, where she works to improve health by accelerating support for medical research through recognition of research excellence, education, and advocacy. As an infectious disease physician, she is passionate about caring for the underserved and addressing the social determinants of health. She is committed to advancing equity and inclusion in science.

She received her BS and MD degrees from the University of Michigan, did residency and fellowship training in infectious disease at the University of Minnesota (U-Minn), and obtained her MBA from the University of Kentucky (U-Kentucky). She has held faculty positions at the U-Minn, U-Kentucky, and University of California, Davis (UC Davis). She became Executive Associate Dean at UC Davis in 2003 and was dean of the School of Medicine and Vice Chancellor for Health from 2005 to 2013.

She served as chair of the AAHC and of the AAMC Council of Deans. She currently serves on the Boards of the Morehouse SOM; Science Philanthropy Alliance; Science Communication Lab; Center for Women in Academic Medicine and Science (CWAMS); Sierra Health Foundation; Haemonetics Corporation; and Embecta Corporation. Dr. Pomeroy was inducted into the National Academy of Medicine in 2011. Among her many honors, she has received honorary degrees from University of Massachusetts SOM (2016) and University of South Florida Morsani SOM (2022).

Dr. Pomeroy has a long track record of mentoring diverse leaders in medicine including currently through CWAMS and the Carol Emmott program.

David N. Bailey, MD, is University of California (UC) San Diego Distinguished Professor of Pathology and Pharmacy Emeritus, Department of Pathology Vice Chair for Education and Academic Affairs, and Deputy Dean of the Skaggs School of Pharmacy & Pharmaceutical Sciences.

At UC San Diego he has been Director of Clinical Laboratories, Department of Pathology Chair, Interim Vice Chancellor for Health Sciences and Dean of the School of Medicine, and Dean for Faculty and Student Matters. At UC Irvine he was Vice Chancellor for Health Affairs and Dean of the School of Medicine.

He received his BS degree in chemistry from Indiana University and his MD degree from Yale University, where he also completed residency and fellowship training in Laboratory Medicine. He is certified in Clinical and Chemical Pathology (American Board of Pathology).

His honors include the Gerald T. Evans Award (Academy of Clinical Laboratory Physicians & Scientists), the UC Regent Edward Dickson Professorship Award, being one of the top ten most cited authors in forensic sciences (1981–1993) (Science Watch), and a UC Presidential Commendation for Distinguished Service. He has served on multiple advisory and governing boards of organizations and health care systems. Several conference rooms at the University and in the San Diego community have been named in his honor.

Over his career David Bailey has mentored hundreds of faculty, trainees, and staff in both formal mentorship programs as well as on an informal basis, and he considers this activity to be one of the most important highlights of his career.

Abbreviations

AAALAC	American Association for Accreditation of Laboratory Animal Care
AAHC	Association of Academic Health Centers
AAMC	Association of American Medical Colleges
ACCME	Accreditation Council for Continuing Medical Education
ACGME	Accreditation Council on Graduate Medical Education
ACS	American College of Surgeons
AHA	American Hospital Association
AHC	Academic Health Center
AI	Artificial/Augmented Intelligence
AMA	American Medical Association
AMC	Academic Medical Center
APT	Appointments, Promotions, and Tenure
CAP	College of American Pathologists
CEO	Chief Executive Officer
CME	Continuing Medical Education
CWAMS	Center for Women in Academic Medicine and Science
DEI	Diversity, Equity, Inclusion
DIO	Designated Institutional Official
DOD	Department of Defense
DOE	Department of Energy
EA	Executive Assistant
ELAM	Executive Leadership in Academic Medicine
FOIA	Freedom of Information Act
GME	Graduate Medical Education
HELP	Harvard Executive Leadership Program
HR	Human Resources
IT	Information Technology
LLC	Limited Liability Corporation
NCI	National Cancer Institute
NGO	Nongovernmental Organization
NIH	National Institutes of Health

NSF	National Science Foundation
PR	Public Relations
RVU	Relative Value Units
SIG	Special Interest Group
SOM	School of Medicine
SWOT	Strengths, Weaknesses, Opportunities, Threats
TJC	The Joint Commission
VP	Vice President

Chapter 1
Introduction

I've just been appointed chair of a medical school department! Now what?

I've led a medical school department for several years and should know all this stuff, but frankly I'm still not sure about some of it and am embarrassed to ask. What do I do?

These are common questions asked by new and experienced department chairs as they try to navigate the challenges and opportunities that are unique to medical schools and their associated academic health centers/academic medical centers (AHC/AMCs). Unlike general university campus department leadership, medical school department chairs usually have a clinical enterprise mission to consider along with the education, research, and university/public service missions common to all departments. In addition, campus department chair positions often rotate among the existing faculty for 5 years or less, while medical school department leaders are frequently recruited from outside the institution and typically serve for 5 years and often longer. The longevity of service coupled with the responsibility of multiple missions tends to give more authority ("power") to medical school department chairs, which is often augmented by the ability to access additional revenue from their clinical, research, and education activities in the health care enterprise.

These factors taken together make the medical school department chair position one of the most complex leadership roles in the school, and indeed the university. While some might feel that leaders of other units (e.g., centers, institutes, clinical programs) face equally daunting tasks, leadership of those units usually involves only one or two focused mission areas. In contrast, medical school department chairs are tasked with multiple missions which they must lead while also having responsibility for the career development and advancement of their faculty and trainees. Moreover, center, institute, and program faculty are usually appointed in medical school departments, thereby creating a complex matrix management process that can further complicate the department chair's job.

Medical school department chairs also must interact with multiple entities (e.g., university, school, medical center). Accordingly, they are faced with issues of alignment, synergy, conflict, and differing priorities among these entities. Given the clinical mission of most medical school departments, they tend to be much larger than many campus departments, creating the need for their chairs to develop a detailed organizational structure to operate the enterprise.

Not surprisingly, department chairs often find themselves handling a large financial operation and feeling that they are more like business executives and managers than academicians and leaders. This can be challenging because many chairs are selected based upon their academic or clinical excellence, which does not necessarily translate into leadership ability [1]. In addition to these complicating factors, department chairs must learn and adapt to the academic and clinical cultures of their institution(s), which can vary substantially from one to another [2] (see Chap. 6).

To be successful, medical school department chairs must be focused on the achievements of their constituents (e.g., faculty, staff, students, trainees), which is confounded by trying to balance their activities in health care delivery with the missions of education, research, and public service. This can be especially difficult because chairs themselves are faculty members, expected to maintain their own academic portfolio as well as perform their leadership and administrative service activities. While challenging, this is not impossible and indeed can provide exciting career directions [3].

As one former chair observed upon stepping down almost 20 years ago, the important issues are many: balancing the budget, serving your unit, leading more and managing less, making time for yourself, encouraging good citizenship by setting an example, developing an appropriate infrastructure, utilizing volunteer faculty, networking, fundraising, and entertaining [4]. While these basic principles are still true, today's medical school department chairs have an even more complex environment due to funding shortfalls, health care disparities, evolving technology, government regulations, and changing workstyles, among many others.

New medical school department chairs are faced with many challenges, the learning curve is steep, some mistakes should be expected, and there often is a lot of on-the-job learning [5]. Not surprisingly, new and even experienced leaders have many questions about how to deal with the problems and opportunities they face every day. This book poses and answers questions commonly asked by department chairs that address major issues including: getting started; setting priorities and running the department; interacting with faculty, staff, students, trainees, institutional leaders, other stakeholders, and external entities; determining and enhancing the skills needed for success; developing a good work-life balance; and dealing with personal concerns.

Finally, it should be noted that while this book focuses on advice for new, experienced, and aspiring medical school department chairs across the many different models that exist for their departments (see Chap. 2, section "Starting Out") [6], many of the suggestions may be helpful for department chairs in other health sciences schools as well as for individuals in other AHC/AMC leadership positions, where many of the issues are similar but may vary in intensity and complexity.

References

1. Gao Z-H. Chairing an academic pathology department: challenges and opportunities. J Clin Pathol. 2019;72:206–12. https://doi.org/10.1136/jclinpath-2017-204963.
2. Sheldon GF. Embrace the challenge: advice for current and prospective department chairs. Acad Med. 2013;88:914–5. https://doi.org/10.1097/ACM.0b013e318294fe01.
3. Zheng EW, Hu J, Levine JS, Ma AC, Guo WA. The catch 22 of promotion: is becoming a department chair of surgery a threat to the triple threat? Surgery. 2022;172:1422–8. https://doi.org/10.1016/j.surg.2022.06.006.
4. Winstead DK. Advice for chairs of academic departments of psychiatry: the "ten commandments". Acad Psychiatry. 2006;30:298–300. https://doi.org/10.1176/appi.ap.30.4.298.
5. Fisher M. Being chair: a 12-step program for medical school chairs. Int J Med Educ. 2011;2:147–51. https://doi.org/10.5116/ijme.4ece.862d.
6. Weiner BJ, Culbertson R, Jones RF, Dickler R. Organizational models for medical school—clinical enterprise relationships. Acad Med. 2001;76:113–24. https://doi.org/10.1097/00001888-200102000-00007.

Part I
Getting Started

One of the most challenging times for any chair is when they are starting in their new position, especially if it is at a new institution. Although there normally is a honeymoon period when beginning, this doesn't diminish the time and effort you need to determine what is expected by the institution and your department, how to deal with your predecessor, how best to communicate your vision and priorities, how to set the initial goals for yourself and your department, and how to enhance your skills to successfully accomplish these expectations. Regardless of your prior experience as a leader or association with the institution, you should expect there will be some unanticipated issues and opportunities, along with good and bad surprises, to deal with early on. Your first steps are important in setting the tone and direction that ultimately will determine your success in leading your department.

Chapter 2
Setting Initial Goals

Starting Out

"What Is the Scope of My Authority and Responsibilities as Chair?"

As a new medical school department chair, it is important to understand how the relationship of your medical school to other parts of your academic health centers/academic medical centers (AHC/AMCs) impacts the scope of your authority and therefore responsibilities, especially in clinical service and training [1]. Several of the different organizational models for medical school departments and the authority of the chair include:

- The medical school department is part of a university that also owns the health system, and the chair is also chief of clinical services in the AHC/AMC.
- The medical school department is part of a university that also owns the health system, but the chair is not the chief of clinical services in the AHC/AMC and may or may not have authority over the chief of clinical services.
- The medical school department is part of a university that does not own the health system, and the chair is also chief of clinical services in the health system.
- The medical school department is part of a university that does not own the health system, and the chair is not the chief of clinical services in the AHC/AMC and may or may not have authority over the chief of clinical services.
- The medical school department is in a free-standing medical college that may or may not control the health system, and the chair may or may not be chief of clinical services in the health system.
- The medical school department is in a free-standing health system, where the chair may or may not be chief of clinical services.

F. Sanfilippo et al., *Lead, Inspire, Thrive*, https://doi.org/10.1007/978-3-031-41177-9_2

For each of these many models, the relationship of your medical school to co-owned, affiliated, or independent healthcare institutions, and of your department to the corresponding clinical specialty service, is the basis for determining your scope of authority and the complexity of your position in interacting with other leaders to fulfill expectations and achieve your department's goals and priorities.

"What Should My "Chair Package" Include?"

Positioning yourself for success as a chair begins before the official first day of your job. Negotiating your "chair package" during the recruitment process is key to ensuring that you will have the resources you need to lead your department forward [2]. In addition to the resources required for your personal and professional success (e.g., compensation, staff support, space, equipment, etc.), it is critical to determine and obtain what the department needs to flourish in the future. By keeping the emphasis on the department [3], you will communicate to institutional leaders and your faculty and staff that your primary goal is the success of the department rather than individual gain.

Determining what you should ask for in your departmental recruitment package starts with clearly formulating and communicating your vision for the department and ensuring that this vision aligns with the institutional goals for the department (see Chap. 30). You should then gather information to understand the resources that will be needed to achieve these expectations and aspirations. Understanding the extent of your authority also is essential to ensure it is properly aligned with your designated responsibilities, so that you will not be held accountable for issues beyond your control.

To negotiate for the appropriate resources, you should understand the finances and current assets in the department, as well as active or anticipated future activities for the department in each mission area. Typically, chair packages include resources for the first 3–5 years. An evidence-based approach to negotiations that focuses on the department's future success signals that you intend to be a team player and assures those to whom you will report that your leadership will advance both the department and the entire AHC/AMC.

Getting advice from others about your chair package can be very helpful. Consider talking with department chairs at your current institution, try to learn about the "norms" for chair packages at your new institution, and listen to your mentors and colleagues who are experienced in such negotiations. The use of national databases to determine benchmarks will augment your evidence base. Remember to keep the agreement for your own professional resources separate from the departmental package, so there is no ambiguity (especially as perceived by faculty and staff) about what is meant for you versus the department.

"What Are the Key Things to Remember as a New Department Chair?"

Starting out as a new department chair is a major transition for you and your department, and your initial days will set the tone for the success of both. Although you will receive a lot of attention as the new leader, it is critical that you focus your attention and priorities on the success of the department rather than on you. This requires that you spend most of your time listening, meeting and engaging stakeholders, forming a leadership team that has the trust and confidence of the department and institution, delegating as much as possible to them so you can focus on the activities that are of major consequence and only you can do, and developing the strategy, vision, goals, and priorities for the future success of your department.

"How Do I Determine What I Need to Know to Fulfill My New Role?"

New leaders come to their positions with varying degrees of experience, ranging from the novice to seasoned individuals. You should carefully evaluate your level of knowledge and confidence in your new role (see Chap. 33) and determine how much and what type of assistance you should seek (see Chap. 34). Above all you should not be embarrassed to ask for help and advice. Wise leaders have enough self-awareness to understand what they know, what they don't know, and especially what they need to know, particularly when starting in a new role.

"What Goals Should I Set for My First 100 Days, Especially If Moving to a New Institution?"

In setting goals, you should place the needs of the department before your own, focus on what you and the institution want your department to accomplish, and remember that the primary responsibility of a leader is the success of their team (i.e., your department). During this initial period, you also may wish to acquire additional skills that may be lacking (e.g., business, management, communication) and incorporate them into personal goal setting (see Chap. 33). Finally, you should have a realistic estimate of the time that you anticipate serving as chair to set an approximate timeline for achieving your goals [4].

The goals set for your first 100 days will lay the foundation for the development of the department under your leadership and will play an important role in how you are viewed by the faculty, the institution, and other constituents. Thus, these goals should be carefully formulated. They should be based upon the results that you and the institution leadership ultimately want to achieve. They should be specific, easily articulated, attainable, measurable, realistic, relevant, and time-based. Importantly, they should be consistent with and reflect the charge you were given during your recruitment and appointment. Faculty and staff acceptance of these goals is essential because it is their achievements that will determine success, which means you should involve them in the process from the outset. In addition, input from students and trainees, as well as community members, and other stakeholders, is usually of great value in getting viewpoints that are important to the mission and often less tied to the status quo.

Setting aggressive but realistic goals for your department to achieve its vision for the future often requires modifying long-standing department practices (see Chap. 12, section "Managing Change"). In an era of increasing changes in research, patient care, and education, effective chairs must be change agents to meet these challenges and opportunities. Accordingly, when setting initial goals, you should evaluate the department to determine what can and should be improved through change. That said, you should not make change just for change's sake. Changes must result in improvements that are measurable and can be understood by your faculty, staff, students, and trainees, as well as institution and community leaders.

An important part of starting out in a new leadership role (as well as throughout your leadership tenure) is to be visible and interactive by walking through the department and meeting faculty, staff, students, and trainees, on their turf, where they are likely to be more comfortable and candid in providing their ideas and feedback. Similarly, visibility and interaction with student and faculty alumni, donors, and other institutional and community stakeholders outside the department will help you learn how your department and the institution work and how they evolved [5].

Clearly, if your vision and goals for the department are too grandiose, they simply will not fly, while if they are too modest they will not add much value. Buy-in and engagement of key constituents is essential in setting goals [6]. While finances need to be considered when developing strategies and tactics, costs should rarely constrain vision because innovative ideas can generate new resources. Once initial goals are set, the department's strategic plan should be reviewed and appropriately revised or replaced to provide the roadmap to achieving those goals (see Chap. 12).

Your Initial Message: First Impressions Are Lasting

"Upon Being Appointed Chair, How and What Should I Communicate to Members of My Department and Institutional Leaders?"

"First impressions are lasting!" Your initial messages will lay the foundation and set the tone for your relationship with the department and institution. Thus, their content and delivery are exceedingly important. Faculty, staff, students, trainees, and institutional leaders often will long remember the first formal address of a new leader.

Initial messages should lay out your goals, vision, and strategy for your department as well as the methods for realizing that vision. They may include discussion of the intended process for determining departmental organizational structure, and for reviewing or developing your department's strategic plan (see Chaps. 11 and 12) [5].

Your initial messaging should also reflect your management style (e.g., being visible and accessible with an "open-door" policy versus meeting by "appointment only"), as well as the communication processes you prefer such as:

- Regularly scheduled faculty meetings
- Divisional meetings
- One-on-one meetings with faculty
- Meetings with staff, students, and trainees
- Publication of a recurring newsletter
- Regular e-mail updates
- Annual department report

Regardless of your preferred style and processes for communication, you should convey your desire to develop a close working relationship with the faculty, staff, students, trainees, and institutional leadership. Since this is a serious time of change for members of your department, adding humor as appropriate to your communication style can help lower anxiety and concern. Joking about your own habits and behaviors is a good way to lessen the distance and facilitate communication between you and members of your department.

"How Should I Communicate Expectations of the Institution to My Department?"

It is essential that department members know what is expected of you and the department. Accordingly, it may be useful for you to share elements of your hiring agreement as they reflect institution expectations, which the faculty, staff, students, and trainees should know. Sharing this information also may help to dispel unrealistic, if not fanciful, notions about the availability of "unlimited" resources that you have been given (see Chap. 13).

In many cases, new department chairs are given resources that extend beyond direct allocations of money and space. In fact, there are many significant opportunities and expectations for your department that might be provided by the institution such as:

- Affiliations
- Approval of new programs
- Alterations in indirect cost recovery policies
- Changes in royalty distribution
- Support of recruitment expenses

Including institution leadership at a faculty meeting may help present a balanced view of what the institution expects of the department, and what resources are being provided to achieve those expectations.

Getting the Faculty and Staff Involved

"How Can I Best Engage My Faculty and Staff in Setting Goals During My First 100 Days?"

Performing a SWOT (strengths, weaknesses, opportunities, and threats) analysis is often an effective means of engaging faculty, staff, and other constituents in the process of setting initial goals. Off-site retreats using professional facilitators may be particularly useful in stimulating thoughts, ideas, and discussion, especially when in an informal and relaxed setting with time for social interactions. Creating workgroups of faculty, staff, students, and trainees to assess issues and opportunities in setting goals is another good way to get them involved. However, their interest in participating probably will be tempered by how much they believe resources actually will be allocated to reach these goals, so your messaging on this point needs to be genuine, clear, and certain.

Getting External Help in Setting Goals

"Whom Should I Involve from Outside the Department to Help Set Initial Goals?"

You may wish to engage outside individuals with expertise in advising, consulting, and/or assessment in setting your initial goals. You also may consider getting advice or assistance to improve the skills you need personally for achieving the goals being set, such as communication and change management. Help already may be available within your institution, or you can hire professional consultants to assist (see Chap. 34).

Your professional societies may be another good source of support because they can help identify trends and themes specific to your department's disciplines. Finally, advice from new and established department chairs at your institution, and peers at other institutions, can be very helpful; there can be a lot to learn from their successes and failures in establishing and ultimately achieving your own initial goals.

References

1. Weiner BJ, Culbertson R, Jones RF, Dickler R. Organizational models for medical school—clinical enterprise relationships. Acad Med. 2001;76:113–24. https://doi.org/10.1097/00001888-200102000-00007.
2. Grigsby RK. Five ways to fail as a new leader in academic medicine. In: Academic physician & scientist. Philadelphia: Lippincott Williams & Wilkins; 2010. p. 4–5. https://adfm.org/media/1036/grigsby_five_ways_to_fail.pdf.
3. Weidner A, Elwood S, Koopman R, Phillips J, Schmitz D, Li L, et al. Negotiating a new chair package: context and considerations. Fam Med Community Health. 2023;11:e002062. https://doi.org/10.1136/fmch-2022-002062.
4. Bailey DN, Buja LM, Gorstein F, Gotlieb A, Green R, Kane A, et al. Life after being a pathology department chair III; reflections on the "afterlife". Acad Pathol. 2019;6:2374289519846068. https://doi.org/10.1177/2374289519846068.
5. Bailey DN, Lipscomb MF, Gorstein F, Wilkinson D, Sanfilippo F. Life after being a pathology department chair II: lessons learned. Acad Pathol. 2017;4:2374289517733734. https://doi.org/10.1177/2374289517733734.
6. Ness RB, Samet JM. How to be a department chair of epidemiology: a survival guide. Am J Epidemiol. 2010;172:747–51. https://doi.org/10.1093/aje/kwq268.

Chapter 3
Expectations

Measuring Your Success

"How Do I Best Determine the Institutional Measures of Success for Me and My Department?"

Measures of success are critical in setting priorities for yourself and your department and should guide what you say, how you plan, how you implement, and how you assess. After meeting and discussing expectations with the individuals to whom you directly report, be sure to get written criteria that will be used for evaluating you personally and your department. For new chairs, this presumably was part of the recruitment process; for established chairs it should be part of an annual review that determines objectives and benchmarks for the year (see Chap. 35) [1].

You should consider using well-accepted criteria for evaluating your own performance and that of your department, which include:

- Academic productivity, grants, and publications
- Community engagement and support
- Evaluations from department faculty
- Evaluations from other administrators and leaders in your institution
- Financial viability and fundraising
- Quality of clinical services
- Quality of educational activities
- Recruitment/retention/diversity of faculty, students, and staff
- Service to the school and university

Remember that as a leader, institutional leaders will measure your personal success in large part by the success of your department and its members!

F. Sanfilippo et al., *Lead, Inspire, Thrive*, https://doi.org/10.1007/978-3-031-41177-9_3

"How Do I Best Determine the Departmental Measures of Success for Me and the Department?"

True excellence of your department requires innovation and productivity on the part of the faculty as well as the success of its students, trainees, and staff. Members of your department will measure success by the accomplishments of the department as a whole and not by your personal achievements [2]. Success will also be measured objectively by your departmental faculty and staff for meeting or exceeding the expectations, goals, and objectives set by institutional leadership.

"How Should I Determine Personal Measures of Success for Me and the Department?"

Your personal measures of success will likely reflect the institutional and departmental expectations mentioned above, as well as your own accomplishments as chair. However, key measures of success should go beyond your leadership achievements and include subjective consideration of what you value and what brings you personal satisfaction. These may include:

- Academic productivity
- Career development
- Community engagement
- Financial stability
- National impact/recognition
- Physical and mental well-being
- Relationships with your supervisors, peers, and those who report to you
- Time with family, friends, and hobbies
- Work-life balance

Input from family, trusted friends, colleagues, and advisors can be very helpful in measuring your personal success and satisfaction (see Chap. 36).

Serving as an Interim Chair

"Should I Consider Serving as an Interim Chair?"

Service as an interim chair can be a useful experience if you potentially are interested in seeking a future chair position [3], or if you wish to make changes that are needed in the department but do not wish to serve as a permanent chair.

Before considering the position of interim chair, you should answer several questions, including:

- Are you able to place the needs of the department first [4]?
- Are you interested in applying for the permanent position?
- Are you willing to put your personal academic and/or clinical productivity at risk knowing that you may not get the permanent position?
- How will you feel if you seek the permanent position and do not get it?
- What are the expectations of the interim chair position?
- What are your personal motives for assuming the position?
- What is the anticipated length of service as interim chair?
- Why did the position become vacant?
- Will the department faculty support you in an interim chair role?

The answer to these questions, with the help of trusted advisors (see Chap. 34), should help you make the best decision.

"How Might Expectations Be Affected If I'm Serving as an Interim Versus a Permanent Chair?"

If appointed as an interim chair, you should explicitly determine with those to whom you report whether your role is primarily as a caretaker (holding the department together during the search for the permanent chair), manager (administering the department without setting the vision and direction), or leader (empowered to make changes and implement your vision and direction). Without this clarification, your activities as an interim chair often will be misunderstood or underappreciated, especially by your faculty and staff.

"Will Expectations About My Role as an Interim Chair Hurt or Improve My Chances of Becoming Permanent Leader?"

If your service as an interim chair is primarily expected to be as a caretaker, you may be viewed as weak and without a personal vision by the department, thereby hurting your chances to become permanent chair. Your chances may also be diminished if expectations are to lead and implement major change and direction, since some faculty and staff who do not like the changes or feel threatened may think that you are overly aggressive and operating outside the boundaries of your authority as interim chair. In either case, it is helpful to have the individuals(s) who appointed you to an interim role meet with the department as a whole to explain the level of your authority and expectations of your role.

The length of time you serve as interim chair can also affect expectations. If your predecessor left unexpectedly, your term of interim leadership is likely to be longer than if your predecessor provided sufficient time for a search to be launched before you were appointed. Although serving longer as an interim chair provides more time to prove yourself, it also gives you more time to make mistakes, disappoint faculty by declining their requests for resources, and exceed your honeymoon period of support.

"Internal" Versus "External" Recruitment

"How Might Expectations Be Affected If I Was an Internal Candidate for the Chair Versus an External Candidate?"

Your prior engagement with the institution as a student, trainee, or faculty member can provide valuable insight about the culture, values, vision, and direction of the department and institution. This can positively affect expectations that you would be able to hit the ground running and launch needed initiatives more quickly than an external candidate. However, your prior relationship can also instill preconceived notions and biases about the department and institution that limit your evaluation of issues. In addition, those involved in your recruitment and appointment also may have preconceived notions about your abilities, priorities, strengths, and weaknesses and believe that external candidates may be more likely to have fresh ideas and different approaches to issues and opportunities.

A common expectation of internal and interim chairs who are candidates for the permanent position is that they will receive fewer resources than an external candidate, which can create a negative perception in the eyes of the department faculty and staff [5]. Ironically, because of the additional resources needed to recruit and relocate external candidates, an internal candidate may actually receive more resources for departmental development. If you are an internal candidate successfully appointed to the chair, try to determine if the resources committed for departmental use would have differed for an external candidate. This can be very helpful in correcting misperceptions that may exist in your department or with peer leaders at the institution.

Prior Leadership Experience

"How Might Expectations Be Affected If I've Previously Served as a Chair?"

The expectations for a lateral move to another institution as chair will be influenced by your reasons for the change, which could be positive (e.g., you accomplished all that was possible and now want additional opportunities) or negative (e.g., you had problems).

Similarly, expectations if you served previously as a chair may be positive based on your accomplishments and experience in dealing with issues and opportunities, or negative based on concerns of your bringing preconceived ways of addressing problems that may not fit the new position. Indeed, in some cases new chairs are chosen primarily for their experience in the same role elsewhere, whereas in other cases, prior service in the same role is considered a liability.

Surprises

"What Should I Watch Out for After Assuming My Role as New Chair?"

Regardless of whether or not one has served as an interim chair in the institution, or even as prior chair at another institution, surprises often occur after assuming your new role. Becoming permanent chair after having served as interim chair may be viewed by some that the institution took the most expeditious route to chair recruitment, which may cast you in a somewhat negative light. This can be offset if a full national search was conducted for the position, and the institution's leaders communicate that your recruitment package was the same as (or perhaps even better than) it would have been for external candidates (see above).

Internal candidates also may be viewed as "pushovers" by their colleagues, particularly those who view them as personal friends and expect to receive favorable treatment as a result. As a new chair you must ensure an objective approach to faculty (as well as staff and students) and avoid even the perception of playing favorites. This may be off-putting to some but is essential for both you and your department's welfare.

If you are a newly appointed chair from the outside, you are likely to discover problems and opportunities that were not apparent to you during interviews. You should realize that this happens to almost every external candidate who is appointed to a leadership position, and simply reflects the fact that one cannot know all the intimate details about a department and institution even after multiple in-depth visits. Ironically, even internal candidates who are appointed chairs often are surprised by institutional policies or practices they did not fully understand, especially at the higher levels of institutional leadership.

Fortunately, there often are as many good as bad surprises for new chairs, but in some cases institutional culture makes the problematic ones much less apparent before assuming the role. Such surprises may cause you to wonder if you made the correct decision in accepting the position of chair. It is important that you remain resilient and do not let surprises overwhelm you as a new chair; there undoubtedly will be more during the course of your leadership.

References

1. Dunning DG, Durham TM, Aksu MN, Lange BM. The state of the art in evaluating the performance of department chairs and division heads. J Dent Educ. 2007;71:467–79. https://doi.org/10.1002/J.0022-0337.2007.71.4.tb04298.x.
2. Willett CG. Reflections from a chair: leadership of a clinical department at an academic medical center. Cancer. 2015;22:3795–8. https://doi.org/10.1002/cncr.29588.
3. Rayburn W, Grigsby K, Brubaker L. The strategic value of succession planning for department chairs. Acad Med. 2016;91:465–8. https://doi.org/10.1097/ACM.0000000000000990.
4. Soltys SM. Primer for the interim chair. Acad Psychiatry. 2011;35:122–5. https://doi.org/10.1176/appi.ap.35.2.122.
5. Bailey DN, George MR, Howell DH, Karcher DS, Libien J, Powell DE, et al. Serving as a temporary pathology chair: "boon" or "boondoggle"? Acad Pathol. 2019;6:2374289519877547. https://doi.org/10.1177/2374289519877547.

Chapter 4
Dealing with Your Predecessor

Developing a Relationship

"How Should I Interact with a Former Chair?"

Interactions with a predecessor are influenced by many factors, especially if you had a prior relationship as colleagues or an appointment in the department when they were the chair. In addition, their success (or lack thereof) as the former chair and continued presence in the department can have significant impact. Regardless of the situation, you should show respect and due consideration to your predecessor, treating them as you would want your successor to treat you [1].

Your department faculty as well as the institutional colleagues of the former chair will take notice of how you interact with the former chair, so it is an opportunity to demonstrate your personality and behavior. As appropriate early after your appointment as chair, it is beneficial to invite departmental faculty, staff, trainees, students, institutional leaders, and key stakeholders to a departmental event that provides recognition and thanks to your predecessor. This can create substantial goodwill and enhance your transition as the new department leader.

In some cases, a new chair knows his/her predecessor as a professional colleague at another institution or as their former chair at the same institution. If you have been professional colleagues, you now have an additional area of potential interaction about department leadership, which can be very helpful. If you were a faculty member in the same department as a former chair who has remained in the department, your prior relationship and interactions are likely to change with the role reversal. Your predecessor may pull back in the relationship to avoid being seen as having too much influence over you, and, accordingly, you may find it difficult to oversee and evaluate your prior chair.

© The Author(s), under exclusive license to Springer Nature
Switzerland AG 2023
F. Sanfilippo et al., *Lead, Inspire, Thrive*,
https://doi.org/10.1007/978-3-031-41177-9_4

If your predecessor was successful and left the institution for a position else-where, it can be very useful to establish a relationship to get advice about the department and institution and especially any issues that contributed to his/her departure.

You should be clear with your predecessor on how you would like to communicate; and agree about when to give and receive advice, assistance, and discuss issues. If the former chair remains in the department, there should be an explicit understanding of your predecessor's role in the department. In some cases, it may be advantageous to give your predecessor a largely honorific title in the department (e.g., "special advisor") to define the boundaries of his/her influence, while giving license to assist you as appropriate [2]. This also may be viewed favorably by the faculty, especially those who supported your predecessor.

Advice and Assistance

"When Should I Ask the Former Chair for Help and Advice?"

The advice and help of a predecessor can be very helpful, especially if they were trusted by the department and institution and were considered successful [3, 4]. It can be exceptionally valuable if you are a new chair from the outside and have issues with individuals they know well and have dealt with in the past, especially with problem faculty and staff, peer institutional leaders, and those who recruited you [1].

If a successful former chair is now at another institution, they may be a bit hesitant to provide help or advice because they are no longer as familiar with the department, especially if you have made significant changes. They also may also feel that it is improper to reinsert themselves into their former department for fear of appearing to interfere.

In the situation where your predecessor has remained at your institution and is now a well-respected faculty member in your department, your past and current interactions will make it clear when and how to ask him/her for help or advice. As appropriate, you should make sure the past chair understands that getting their advice does not imply that they have decision rights or veto power on issues. Likewise, in some cases you should get their advice and help in a confidential manner, so that others do not infer that your predecessor is still running the department or that you are unable to make decisions [5].

Dealing with Interference

"How Should I Deal with Problems Created by My Predecessor?"

This is a special case of dealing with problem faculty in your department (see Chap. 20) and should be handled with extreme care because of the substantial risk to reputations and relationships (both yours, your predecessor, and others). Remember that former chairs likely will have developed relationships with a broad range of internal and external stakeholders, whom they may engage to pressure you.

Problems with former chairs can include excessive demands for resources, open resistance or even frank opposition to your initiatives, and covert attempts to subvert your authority, reputation, or relationships with faculty, peers, supervisors, alumni, donors, or community leaders whom they know well.

Former chairs demanding inappropriate support or resources generally should be handled with the same due consideration as with other faculty. Of course, if the institution made commitments to the former chair in their transition, those commitments must be honored.

In many cases, unsuccessful former chairs who were removed or who "voluntarily" resigned will express anger or revenge by not supporting their successor, especially if it is someone who was in their department and did not support them while they were the chair. Fortunately, this behavior is usually transparent and their ability to cause problems is mitigated by their poor past performance and removal from the position. Nonetheless, such former chairs can create many problems and should be watched and dealt with carefully. They also are more likely to be disruptive and even litigious if they were forced to step down.

Unfortunately, in some cases even successful former chairs cannot deal with losing the authority and position they had previously and may show opposition to any changes you make because they feel it is an insult to their past leadership or they are trying to retain control. However, if you focus on emphasizing your commitment to the department's mission and the importance of broad engagement of all stakeholders, you will gain the confidence of the department and maybe even win over a skeptical predecessor.

References

1. Fisher M. Being chair: a 12-step program for medical school chairs. Int J Med Educ. 2011;2:147–51. https://doi.org/10.5116/ijme.4ece.862d.
2. Bailey DN, Lipscomb MF, Gorstein F, Wilkinson D, Sanfilippo F. Life after being a pathology department chair: issues and opportunities. Acad Pathol. 2016;3:2374289516673651. https://doi.org/10.1177/2374289516673651.

3. Bailey DN, Cohen S, Gotlieb A, Lipscomb MF, Sanfilippo F. What advice current pathology chairs seek from former chairs. Acad Pathol. 2018;5:2374289518807397. https://doi.org/10.1177/2374289518807397.
4. Sanfilippo F, Markwood P, Bailey DN. Retaining the value of former department chairs: the association of pathology chairs experience. Acad Pathol. 2020;7:2374289520981685. https://doi.org/10.1177/2374289520981685.
5. Bailey DN, Buja LM, Gorstein F, Gotlieb A, Green R, Kane A, et al. Life after being a pathology department chair III: reflections on the "afterlife". Acad Pathol. 2019;6:2374289519846068. https://doi.org/10.1177/2374289519846068.

Part II
Interpersonal Interactions, Culture, and Behavior

Successful leadership requires the ability to engage and motivate members of your team to create a constructive, collaborative, collegial, diverse, inclusive, and achievement-oriented culture. Your interactions with stakeholders set a tone for your department, and your behavior should be a role model for those you lead. The style and skill of your communication in speech, words, and actions is the basis for productive interactions and can enhance achievement of your goals. The success of your leadership is highly dependent on effectively communicating a commitment to excellence in all the department's missions; the importance of diversity, equity, and inclusion; the ways that collaboration, collegiality, teamwork, and negotiation can create value; and the benefits of a healthy work-life balance. The organizational culture and behavioral norms you promote will have a major impact on the performance and success of you and your department.

Chapter 5
Communication

Enhancing Your Communication Skills

"How Can I Improve My Speaking Skills?"

All chairs have substantial experience speaking to the students they teach and train, as well as colleagues in their scientific field of study or clinical practice. However, speaking as a leader on subjects and to people outside your discipline can be a significant challenge and requires additional skills. This especially comes into play when trying to motivate faculty and staff about strategy, tactics, and priorities for achieving departmental goals and the expectations of your institution. Moreover, a leadership communication style that may be effective with your students or professional colleagues is not necessarily the right approach with other stakeholders (e.g., donors, the media, etc.; see Chap. 31).

A key to effective communication is adapting to your audience (i.e., providing context and making connections while telling them what they need to hear). You should try to tailor your communication to what they already know about the topic by adjusting the background and details you provide, as well as considering the specialized language and jargon you should or should not use. Moreover, it is helpful to anticipate their own interests and feelings about the topic you are discussing, especially if you are trying to explain a new issue or get their cooperation and support.

Making your presentation to an audience more like a conversation rather than a speech usually will increase their attention and understanding of the message you are trying to deliver. Listening and striving to understand and consider the audience's perspectives is key to effective communication. And always remember that what you say or write often will be interpreted differently by individuals who vary in age, race, ethnicity, native language, and other characteristics.

© The Author(s), under exclusive license to Springer Nature Switzerland AG 2023

F. Sanfilippo et al., *Lead, Inspire, Thrive*,

https://doi.org/10.1007/978-3-031-41177-9_5

Communication is an art and a science, and even the best communicators can learn from instructors and improve with coaching. A good first step for improving your skills as a speaker is to get an objective evaluation by experts. As is often the case, you may be completely unaware of subtle features of your body language, intonation, or manner of hesitation that can have a significant impact on your effectiveness in speaking with an individual or presenting to an audience. Your institutional communications staff can help in this process or refer you to the appropriate resources. The time spent to become a more effective speaker, especially in group and public settings, can be of tremendous benefit by increasing your ability to accurately transmit your intended thoughts and messages. Moreover, by improving your comfort and confidence while speaking, audiences are more likely to believe what you tell them and support your position on issues being discussed.

"How Can I Improve My Writing Skills?"

Similar to speaking skills, your experience in writing papers, grants, or reports in your areas of expertise may not be of much help in the writing required for your role as a leader. Being able to write in a manner that is clear and easily understood by a diverse audience of stakeholders requires substantial skill and talent, whether writing an annual review letter to a faculty member or an article explaining the vision and goals of your department to the broad readership of an institutional publication.

As with speaking, an evaluation of your writing skills and style can be very helpful in identifying ways to improve your effectiveness. A key tenet for effective writing, as with speaking, is to anticipate what your recipient or audience expects and needs to understand, so you can express yourself to address those expectations. Simple tricks on how to position words in a sentence, sentences in a paragraph, and paragraphs in a document can substantially help provide the right emphasis and clarity of your message [1]. Perhaps of greatest value is having expert communications staff available who can provide candid feedback and help to draft, review, advise, or edit your correspondence as appropriate. Access to good communication resources can save you substantial time and anxiety, as well as increase your effectiveness.

"How and When Should I Use Different Types of Communication?"

Effective leadership starts with communication [2]. Your preferred method of communication will largely depend upon its relative urgency, the complexity of the message to be transmitted, the audience to be contacted (individual versus group), and the need for documentation or confidentiality.

Urgent messages are best conveyed with a telephone call or text, but if urgent messages are for several individuals, then a quickly convened meeting may be best, which can be virtual or in-person depending on the circumstances. If the subject matter is complex, or you are dealing with a personal issue, it is best to convey it verbally via a meeting or phone call to allow for the time and discourse needed to be sure the message is understood. Similarly, it is best to transmit a confidential message in person or by phone to avoid sending written documents, which may be subject to disclosure under various circumstances.

For communication of nonurgent and nonconfidential items, an e-mail or written note is often best, which will allow more time for a thoughtful response. In-person meetings may be appropriate when you desire more opportunities for interaction, but must be weighed against the added time commitment of the participants. As discussed in Chap. 11 (section "Meetings and Events"), meeting overload is a significant problem not just for you but also for many of your faculty and staff. Fortunately, the much greater use of virtual meetings in the past few years has made this a useful option.

When you wish to document communications with others, e-mail is probably the most reliable, most rapid, and most efficient method to use. However, the abundance of e-mails received by most people today creates considerable uncertainty about whether your e-mail will be received, filtered into junk mail, or inadvertently deleted and, even if received, whether it will be read and acted upon. Generally speaking, if a response is expected but not returned promptly from e-mail recipients, it is prudent to follow up with them to ensure that the communication was indeed received.

Finally, handwritten or typed letters should be used when conveying personal recognition (e.g., for outstanding achievements) and gratitude (e.g., for donations, participation in events, personal assistance), particularly if the recipient is outside of your institution or an important member of your leadership team.

"How Much Should I Read into Body Language?"

Body language at in-person meetings can help convey information, particularly regarding confidence and enthusiasm, and sometimes you can gauge receptivity (both positive and negative) of your audience when messages are delivered face-to-face. However, it often is difficult to correctly read body language; in-person assessments of an issue sometimes can be less accurate than a simple and objective evaluation of the data and information at hand.

You should always be careful if a personal interaction suggests changing the conclusions you would otherwise make, especially when negotiating, considering issues with problem faculty, students, or staff, and when meeting with individuals from a different background. Misinterpretation of body language or unconscious bias may inappropriately influence your assessment [3].

It is important to remember that when speaking, if your words say one thing but your body language says another, your message may be confusing or misinterpreted. This is important to remember when speaking before groups, where a wide range of interpretations of body language (as well as your spoken words) can be made by different listeners.

Transparency and Establishing Trust

"How Can I Best Maintain Communication to Establish Trust and Confidence?"

The effectiveness of your communication to stakeholders has a significant impact on their engagement, trust, and confidence. The heart of good communication is transparency, authenticity, and honesty. Professional experts may be helpful in improving your personal and written communication effectiveness, especially in dealing with complex or controversial issues (see Chap. 34).

Meetings with faculty and staff are especially important venues for disseminating information. Faculty meetings, as well as occasional department-wide "town halls" should be regular events and begin early in your tenure as chair. Faculty and staff want to be recognized for their accomplishments, and such meetings are important opportunities to announce particularly noteworthy achievements. Every meeting also should include an "open forum" to permit participants to introduce any issues they wish. Topics that are particularly sensitive or require background research should be scheduled for discussion at a subsequent meeting after appropriate data and information are gathered. It is also important to admit when you don't know the answer to a question or about information on a topic raised, and to indicate that you will investigate and follow up.

To facilitate intra-departmental alignment and interdisciplinary opportunities, you should schedule faculty meetings that include presentations from different sections of the department to provide updates on their clinical, research, education, and outreach activities and programs (see Chap. 8). Departmental publications and newsletters are additional ways to inform faculty, staff, trainees, and students about the activities underway in different parts of the department. Likewise, scheduling informal tours ("leading by walking around") to visit various groups and programs in your department can be very helpful in learning about their activities and being visible and approachable as a leader.

It is important to respond to all e-mails, texts, and notes even if it is only to acknowledge their receipt with a simple "thank-you." Ideally you should respond promptly or within the same day whenever possible. Otherwise, faculty and staff will not be sure if you have read their e-mail and may even think that you are ignoring them or do not appreciate their comments. To ensure that you have not overlooked e-mails requiring responses, you should review e-mails at the end of each day or have a trusted assistant do so.

The establishment of a department "executive committee" consisting of key program, administrative, and thought leaders in the department is also an effective method of communication and can be used as a sounding board for your ideas prior to presentation to internal or external groups. Such a committee also increases consistency in messaging among your lieutenants and administrative staff and can provide backup support if they have endorsed proposals you have made that are considered unpopular or controversial.

"How Do I Promote Feedback and Constructive Advice from My Department and Institutional Leaders?"

You should actively solicit input, feedback, and advice from faculty and institutional leadership and always show your gratitude and appreciation for the gift of receiving candid feedback and advice [4]. If not already in place, you should ask for an annual written evaluation of your personal performance as well as the performance of your department from those to whom you report, which should include input from your department (see Chap. 35). To help promote feedback and advice, you should network throughout the institution to clearly communicate your departmental mission, values, and expectations (see Chaps. 28 and 29) [5].

Many faculty, staff, trainees, and students may be hesitant to bring problems, requests, or advice to you directly, especially if you are new and from another institution, so having lieutenants that they are comfortable approaching can be a great asset. Perhaps most importantly, finding a senior staff or faculty member who is trusted by faculty to serve as a formal or informal "chief of staff" can help immensely in facilitating messaging and communication between you and members of your department. Likewise, your personal executive assistant (EA) is an important point of contact and communication for you and should be someone that is well trusted and easily approachable by those within and outside your department.

"How Should I Deal with Gossip and Rumors About Departmental and Institutional Leaders and Their Decisions?"

Unfortunately, because of visibility and influence, leaders in most organization are often the subject of gossip and rumors, which can involve assumptions about them personally (e.g., leaving for a better position or being fired or disciplined) and decisions they have made or plan to make (e.g., new policies or change in priorities). Dealing with gossip and rumors is difficult, especially since so many are completely inaccurate and often negative.

There are several things to consider in dealing with gossip, particularly their source, accuracy, and apparent intent. As chair, it is likely that you will hear about negative gossip only from your most trusted lieutenants who are comfortable informing you that rumors are being spread; nevertheless, they may be reluctant to reveal (or are unaware of) the primary source. Some rumors are not contrived or meant to be harmful, but rather are an informal means of communicating what is thought to be factual, beneficial, and of interest. Such "positive gossip" can actually reflect healthy engagement and teamwork among members of the department.

The first step in dealing with inaccurate or malicious gossip is to face the source, usually through the lieutenant that reported it, and make it clear that such behavior is unacceptable in an organization that values collegiality. Inaccurate facts also should be asked to be corrected. This can also be an opportunity to connect with the person and try to understand their true motivation for the behavior. Avoid addressing gossip and rumors with broad announcements, which can be counter-productive by making them seem credible and cause potential concern and questions from those who had not heard the gossip or rumors.

"How Should I Handle Freedom of Speech and Academic Freedom Issues That May Come Up?"

The First Amendment guarantees the right to free expression and free association, but with limits on speech that is considered obscene, defamatory, threatening, or inciting physical harm or criminal conduct. Further, academic freedom is a basic tenet at universities. Academic freedom is the right of faculty to express their ideas and opinions without censorship, threat to their tenure or appointment, or institutional retaliation, but with limits on imposing their views on students and requiring compliance with policies and laws against harassing, threatening, intimidating, or ridiculing others.

Since there is often debate and nuance on what is or is not allowed, what appears to be inappropriate and clearly offensive speech to some may be considered by others to be protected under freedom of speech or academic freedom. When such controversies arise with faculty, staff, students, or trainees in your department, it is important to determine if the speech in question is indeed protected and, if not, handle the situation quickly and appropriately as per your institutional policies (see Chaps. 20, 23, and 27).

If speech considered offensive by some is protected, enlist experienced experts [e.g., Human Resources (HR) staff, legal counsel, etc.] to interact with all sides on the underlying principles of free speech and academic freedom, as well as the potential misinterpretations of the intent or inference of the speech, the need for greater sensitivity to the feelings of others, especially those with different backgrounds or beliefs (see Chap. 7), and understanding the significant damage such speech can cause on collegiality, collaboration, trust, and culture (see Chaps. 6 and 8).

Principles of negotiation sometimes can be helpful in bringing sides together (see Chap. 10), and being prepared to deal with the media is well advised (see Chap. 31, section "The Media").

Accommodating Institutional Priorities and Reforms

"How Do I Communicate Institutional Priorities and Decisions to My Faculty and Staff, Especially When I Personally Disagree with Them?"

Although you may disagree personally with an institutional priority or decision, as an institutional leader your responsibility is to develop a way to be supportive. You should communicate to your department the various perspectives the institution's leadership considered, why they made their decision, and why those decisions and priorities should be supported by the department as part of the institution. After an institutional decision is made and agreed upon, it is unwise to publicly or even privately state that you disagree with the decisions or the leaders who made them, as it will reflect poorly on you by creating ambiguity with your department and likely will get back to the institutional leaders. At all costs, you must avoid creating conflict between the department and the institution.

The time for you to disagree with an institutional priority or decision is when it is being discussed and considered, not after a decision is made. Such disagreements during decision-making always should include constructive, viable alternatives and consider potential unintended consequences. As an institutional team player, communicate disagreements in the manner you would want your own team members to communicate a decision you made with which they disagreed.

"How Do I Advocate for My Department During Institutional Reallocation of Resources, Curriculum Changes, Etc.?"

The best way to advocate for your department is by documenting with data the contributions that your department can make to facilitate the proposed changes. Collaboration with other units may be helpful in this regard. In full transparency, and as a true institutional team player, you also should consider what opportunity costs and losses the institution may incur, and how those costs or losses may affect the welfare of your department, and then communicate them objectively and dispassionately to institutional leadership.

"How Do I Best Prepare My Faculty for a Significant Change in the Department, School, University, or AHC/AMC?"

Communicating significant changes affecting the department, particularly those involving reallocation of resources and priorities, is among the most difficult issues you will face as chair. Effective communication can help your faculty and staff understand the rationale for the changes and address their concerns. It may be helpful to invite institutional leaders to meet with the department to explain the reasons for the proposed changes and to hear the potential effects on the department which, in turn, may impact the institution. It also will give your department members the opportunity to hear first-hand from institutional leaders and provide them with direct feedback. Although faculty do not like to hear bad news, they can better accept it if they are engaged at some point in the discussion.

References

1. Gopen G. The sense of structure: writing from the reader's perspective. London: Pearson; 2006. ISBN 978-205296323.
2. Cunningham L. A toolkit for improving communication in your healthcare organization. Front Health Serv Mgmt. 2019;36:3–13. https://doi.org/10.1097/HAP.0000000000000066.
3. Gladwell M. Talking to strangers. Boston: Little, Brown and Company; 2019. ISBN 978-0316478576.
4. Sanfilippo F, Powell D, Folberg R, Tykocinski M. Dealing with deans and academic medical center leadership: advice from leaders. Acad Pathol. 2018;5:2374289518765462. https://doi.org/10.1177/2374289518765462.
5. Winstead DK. Advice for chairs of academic departments of psychiatry: the "ten commandments". Acad Psychiatry. 2006;30:298–300. https://doi.org/10.1176/appi.ap.30.4.298.

Chapter 6
Organizational Culture

Understanding Culture Types and Styles

"What Do I Need to Know About Organizational Culture?"

The culture of your department essentially represents the norms of faculty, staff, trainee, and student behavior and interactions. Culture is strongly related to values and can enhance or completely disrupt strategic plans and priorities. Peter Drucker, one of the greatest of all management consultants, is often quoted for saying "culture eats strategy for breakfast" [1].

It also is important to realize that different sections of your department may have different behavioral norms (culture), which often reflect differences in the leadership of those units. The same is true for different departments at your institution.

The culture of an organization is closely tied to the values, expectations, and direction of the leader, which is why you likely will be held accountable for the culture of your department. The culture(s) in your department also may be affected by external factors, such as regional geopolitical influences, and whether the organization is public (with full disclosure of personnel information including salaries, position descriptions, etc.) or private (with fewer requirements for transparency) [2].

"What Are the Different Culture Types and Styles of Which I Should Be Aware?"

There are several different systems that describe cultural styles and types. A simple and common approach is to characterize culture into three overall types: passive, aggressive, and constructive. In addition to these general types of culture are many specific styles, which in different combinations account for each of these general

F. Sanfilippo et al., *Lead, Inspire, Thrive*, https://doi.org/10.1007/978-3-031-41177-9_6

types. For example, culture styles of achievement, innovation, and collaboration are strongly associated with constructive types of culture, while avoidance and dependency styles are more associated with passive cultures, and competitive, oppositional styles more with aggressive cultures [3].

Organizations with a dominant constructive culture are typically the most satisfying in which to work. They tend to have the highest overall performance and greatest adaptability. Leaders of departments with a constructive culture have an easier time engaging members, making decisions, and initiating changes. Departments with a dominant aggressive culture can be very high performing but tend to have more turf battles. Leaders of departments with a dominant aggressive culture often receive lots of feedback with criticism, have a more difficult time getting consensus on goals and priorities, and find it harder to develop teamwork. Departments with a dominant passive culture tend to have a pleasant environment but members are less transparent, more risk averse, and generally satisfied with the status quo. Leaders of departments with a dominant passive culture have a harder time getting candid feedback, engaging members, and implementing change.

Evaluating Your Organizational Culture(s)

"How Can I Evaluate the Culture of My Department?"

The best way to evaluate the culture(s) of your department is to look at both internal and external manifestations. Personal interactions with faculty, staff, trainees, and students in your department can provide a reasonable sense of their behavioral norms and values, and obtaining input from those outside the department who interact with members extensively can provide important confirmation of your internal assessment.

Depending on the situation, you also may want to make a detailed and objective evaluation of your departmental culture, especially if there is need for change. There are assessment tools that have been shown to be useful in determining organizational culture types and styles in companies as well as AHCs/AMCs [3, 4]. However, the process of using such tools in surveying your faculty and staff should be done carefully, transparently, rigorously, and with the engagement of your institutional HR department. In conducting any culture assessment, it is essential that all participants understand the process being used, and that all responses will be kept strictly confidential from you and other members of the department to avoid bias and conflicts.

"How Do I Determine If the Culture in My Department Needs to Change?"

In the course of being recruited, you should have developed a sense of the culture of your department and how it is viewed by the institution's leaders. In particular, you should have determined or been told if it needs overall improvement or perhaps improvement in some units. An important way to determine if the culture needs to change is by assessing the satisfaction level of your faculty, staff, trainees, and students, as well as your institution's leaders, with the current norms and expectations of behavior. This can be done informally or objectively by rigorous survey as part of a culture assessment of your department.

Driving Culture Change

"How Can I Improve the Culture of My Department?"

The ability to change culture to more constructive styles has been well demonstrated in business organizations and shown to be associated with changes in performance, productivity, and job satisfaction in AHCs/AMCs [4]. However, changing and improving the culture of your department should not be taken lightly; it is a difficult process requiring years of work and your direct oversight and leadership.

There are several keys to leading culture change in your department. One of the most important is to know your department's current culture and the changes desired, since the change process can vary greatly depending on its baseline culture types and styles. Another key is taking personal ownership of the process and being transparent about the rationale, goals, and ongoing metrics to be used in measuring the baseline culture and the changes expected over time.

Perhaps the most important key to success is getting broad support and engagement of your faculty, staff, trainees, and students in the process by explaining how the improvement in culture will create a better and more productive work environment. This can help overcome resistance, especially if baseline assessments show that they are dissatisfied with the current culture. Because of the complexity and high risks (and rewards) in trying to change culture, it is essential to get help in the process from experts in the field, such as from external consultants and your own institutional HR department.

Promoting Teamwork

"How Can I Develop and Improve Teamwork in My Department?"

As mentioned above, good teamwork among faculty and staff reflects a constructive culture with attributes of cooperation, communication, and collaboration that impact overall performance and personal satisfaction. With the significant expansion of knowledge and technology over the past few decades, productivity in research, education, health-care delivery, and community service and outreach all have become more team-oriented. However, most faculty rewards and recognition (e.g., promotion, awards, compensation) have remained focused on individual achievements such as being the principal investigator on grants and the first or senior author on publications.

A key to success in promoting teamwork is demonstrating how it can benefit individual members of the team as well as the department and institution overall [5]. It is very useful to provide examples of how being part of a team can help an individual's career development by enhancing their productivity, creating more professional and administrative opportunities, and at the same time allowing more focus on their individual expertise as part of the team. Likewise, utilizing programs that detail the value of teamwork can be very helpful, especially ones that include practical exercises demonstrating increased performance and satisfaction for team participants. In some cases, analogies to sport teams, acting casts, or orchestras can provide useful examples for explaining good teamwork, especially in describing the value of individuals playing different roles to provide the best overall performance for the department.

Your personal actions are critical in promoting teamwork for your faculty, staff, and students/trainees. This includes developing rewards and incentives for good team players and their teams and by serving as a positive role model for teamwork through your own leadership and professional activities. In particular, it is important to demonstrate that you are a good team player on your institution's teams and a good team leader on your department's teams.

References

1. Drucker P. The effective executive: the definitive guide to getting the right things done. New York: Harper Business; 2006. ISBN 978-0060833459.
2. Fisher M. Being chair: a 12-step program for medical school chairs. Int J Med Educ. 2011;2:147–51. https://doi.org/10.5116/ijme.4ece.862d.
3. Sanfilippo F, Bendapudi N, Rucci A, Schlesinger L. Strong leadership and teamwork drive culture and performance change: Ohio State University Medical Center 2000-2006. Acad Med. 2008;83:845–54. https://doi.org/10.1097/ACM.0b013e318181d2e7.

4. Sanfilippo F, Burns KH, Borowitz ML, Jackson JB, Hruban RH. The Johns Hopkins Department of Pathology novel organizational model: a 25-year ongoing experiment. Acad Pathol. 2018;5:2374289518811145. https://doi.org/10.1177/2374289518811145.
5. Sanfilippo F, Powell D, Folberg R, Tykocinski M. Dealing with deans and academic medical center leadership: advice from leaders. Acad Pathol. 2018;5:2374289518765462. https://doi.org/10.1177/2374289518765462.

Chapter 7
Diversity, Equity, and Inclusion

Highlighting the Importance of Diversity, Equity, and Inclusion (DEI)

"How Can I Highlight the Importance of DEI for My Department?"

Diversity is a key driver of excellence. Extensive research has documented that diverse teams reach better decisions and achieve better outcomes than nondiverse groups [1]. As chair, you should highlight these findings and encourage diversity as a powerful way to achieve excellence. Ensuring input from diverse constituencies requires an inclusive organizational culture in which everyone believes that their input is respected and valued. Clear messages about the unacceptability of harassment and bias are the foundation for the development of truly inclusive workplaces, learning environments, and care delivery.

Persistent realities of pay inequities, disparities in allocation of space and other resources, biased evaluations, stereotyped assignments, microaggressions, overt harassment, and discrimination remain for women and those from groups historically excluded from academic medicine. Chairs who recognize and articulate these historical and ongoing barriers to success send powerful messages about the department's culture to all its members.

Part of prioritizing DEI as an integral part of your department's culture is to discuss its importance in facilitating collaboration and collegiality (see Chap. 8), as well as benefiting the organizational culture and programmatic excellence of the department (see Chap. 6). Embracing the importance of DEI in all the department's missions can advance clinical, education, research, and community service programs. For example, the department's clinical work should include assessment of how well the programs promote health equity, including evaluation of outcomes

© The Author(s), under exclusive license to Springer Nature Switzerland AG 2023

F. Sanfilippo et al., *Lead, Inspire, Thrive*,
https://doi.org/10.1007/978-3-031-41177-9_7

analyzed by gender, geography, race/ethnicity, socioeconomic status, and other parameters, often with the use of tools such as a health equity scorecard [2].

Incorporating DEI in curriculum and training opportunities broadens classroom discussions and prepares trainees to work more effectively in diverse cultural settings (see Chap. 22). Consideration of DEI in research initiatives helps ensure that findings are more applicable to all patients, for example, by ensuring that diverse patient populations are represented in clinical trials. Further, these and other benefits enhance faculty, staff, and trainee productivity and morale (see Chaps. 18, 22, and 25) and therefore personal and departmental success.

As chair, how you model the values of your department and your attention to DEI issues will be closely watched by faculty, staff, trainees, students, and members of the community. You should articulate your commitment to DEI in your communications as well as actively "live" it through your behavior on an interpersonal level, with recommended policies and practices, and by the implementation of programs.

DEI Education and Training

"What Are the Best Ways to Provide Training About DEI in My Department?"

Training programs about DEI, cultural competency, and anti-racism recently have been implemented widely and range from online modules to self-assessment tools, lectures, and more. You should become familiar with the required and optional training programs provided by your institution and then determine additional strategies that address the needs of faculty, staff, trainees, and students in your department. Providing DEI educational content in discussion formats that engage participants such as forums, interest group meetings, workshops, retreats, and symposia is superior to more passive "talking head" lectures. It also is important to provide and discuss appropriate publications and studies as part of an evidence-based departmental educational program on DEI and cultural competency.

There are many publications that can contribute to evidence-based DEI training. These resources highlight the need for greater emphasis on DEI in medical education, research design, and clinical practice to mitigate the long history of bias and discrimination based on race, gender, religion, sexual orientation, socioeconomic status, disability, and ethnicity [3–6]. For example, studies have found that challenges for potential women leaders in academic medicine [7–13] may include feeling unprepared for the role; having a limited number of role models and mentors [9]; having too heavy a clinical burden and lack of time, training, and/or funding to pursue research [10]; and hierarchal issues (e.g., indeterminate tenure of department leaders, allowing for few vacancies over time) [7]. One study reported that women leaders tend to be in smaller departments and tend to have a clinical or educational rather than a research focus [13].

Additional publications are available that focus on historically excluded and under-represented groups in faculty and leadership positions [14–17]. For students and trainees, studies show that despite the expanded number of schools the number of Black men and the number of Native Americans in medical school today remains comparable to the number enrolled four decades ago [18]. This remains true despite documented improved provider-patient communication and in some cases better outcomes when care is provided by gender-, race- and language-congruent providers [19, 20] and the observation that physicians from underrepresented groups are more likely to practice in medically underserved and primary health professional shortage areas [21].

Enhancing and Promoting DEI

"How Do I Promote and Enhance DEI in My Department?"

In addition to the DEI educational programs that you can provide for your department, you should recognize the challenges that bias and discrimination present to your faculty, staff, trainees, and students, and attempt to address these in the working and learning environments of your department and institution. Most schools, hospitals, and institutions have a leader such as a vice dean, vice president (VP), or vice chancellor who oversees DEI and who monitors progress in these areas. You should seek advice and resources from this leader and consider appointing an appropriate individual to oversee DEI activities in your department who is well recognized as strongly committed to DEI by members of your department and the institution.

To demonstrate the importance of DEI to you and the faculty, staff, trainees, and students in your department, the department DEI leader who you appoint should report to you directly and be a member of your executive team. However, it is critical for you as chair to be personally and actively engaged in the DEI activities in your department and institution. Despite the existence of a position/office for DEI in your department and in the institution, as chair you should emphasize and personally demonstrate that DEI must be the responsibility of everyone.

"How Do I Ensure That Departmental Practices Support Recruitment of Diverse Candidates?"

An obvious means of enhancing diversity is recruitment—for faculty, staff, students, and trainees (see Chaps. 17, 21, and 24). For faculty and staff, attention should be paid to the recruitment notice to eliminate unconscious bias in the description and selection criteria. Best practices for searches include ensuring diverse representation on the search committee, educating all committee members about unconscious and other forms of bias, and requirements for diverse candidate slates. Utilization of a search firm can often help identify diverse prospective applicants. In addition, institution recruitment officers can assist you and your department in improving diversity.

"What Are Best Practices for Enhancing an Inclusive and Equitable Culture in My Department?"

Of course, policies that prohibit harassment and discrimination must be strictly enforced. To be effective, supportive, "safe" ways for those who experience these behaviors to report the transgressions must be in place, included in orientation materials, and reinforced regularly. It can be a risky act for someone to report misconduct, and as chair you should ensure that anyone who does so is protected and supported.

As mentioned, most institutions have programs and courses available to improve equity and inclusion awareness, such as training to address implicit bias and cultural competency. These areas also can be a focus for the educational activities developed in your department (see above). Faculty, staff, trainees, and students should be encouraged to increase their awareness of existing biases by using validated measures such as the Implicit Association Test (IAT) as well as reflection and identity exercises [22].

An inclusive and equitable department must have policies and practices that ensure equity in pay, resource allocation, assignments, committee responsibilities, career development opportunities, leave policies, and more. As chair, you should assess decisions about the workplace, research, and learning environments to ensure that a DEI lens has been applied to help make the best choices.

Many other activities can enhance a culture of inclusiveness. Departmental celebrations of special holidays (e.g., Martin Luther King Day) and designated events (e.g., Women in Medicine Month, Minority Health Month) reflect the values of your organization. Recognition events that highlight outstanding achievements of faculty, staff, trainees, and students who are women or from underrepresented groups can provide important role models. Chairs should ensure that invited speakers or guest faculty in their department include experts from diverse groups. In addition, participation in community events that are sponsored by the diverse constituencies served by your department helps build awareness and trust.

It is important to remember that DEI issues extend throughout the department, the school, and the AHC/AMC as a whole, affecting students, trainees, staff, faculty, and administration. DEI should be a significant component of your department's (and institution's) strategic plans, which should address compensation, recruitment and advancement, and evidence-based and standardized approaches to eliminate/mitigate bias [23] and encourage authentic inclusion.

"How Can Career Development Programs Help Advance DEI in My Department?"

Career development programs can support women and those from underrepresented groups to excel in their faculty, staff, trainee, or student role (see Chaps. 18, 22, and 25). Chairs should consider providing time and using department funds to support faculty participation in career development programs and familiarize themselves with career development opportunities available at their own institution and nationally.

A number of medical schools have designed programs that offer a combination of experiences specifically focused on women or members of under-represented groups, plus experiences that bring together those with differing life experiences. Additional options include courses such as those offered by Drexel University's Executive Leadership in Academic Medicine (ELAM) [24] and the AAMC, and conferences sponsored by groups such as the National Hispanic Medical Association and the National Medical Association, among others. Mentoring and executive coaching can also be career- and life-changing. An array of mentoring programs are available, both locally and nationally, such as the Carol Emmott Fellowship [25] and the Faculty Advising Network of the Center for Women in Academic Medicine and Science (CWAMS) [26].

"How Do I Avoid Exacting 'Gender or Minority Taxes'?"

Frequently women and those from underrepresented groups are disproportionately called upon to represent or advocate for their communities. The resulting burden on their time and resources has been termed "gender" and "minority" taxes [27, 28]. These responsibility disparities occur when organizations disproportionately expect or rely upon those from underrepresented groups to play service roles, often with the aim of ensuring "representation" of diversity. In academic medicine, this can include inequitable committee service burdens, requests for mentorship, clinical responsibilities especially those aimed at underserved patients, DEI activities, and community engagement. Because of the smaller numbers of faculty, staff, trainees, and students from these groups, they are often repeatedly asked to take on these roles, many of which do not directly advance their career development. Chairs should ensure that such activities are fairly distributed so that all department members have the opportunity to achieve their maximum career growth and satisfaction.

Measuring Success

"How Should I Monitor DEI in My Department?"

Since activities that are not measured are assumed to be unimportant, you should utilize specific metrics to monitor progress in enhancing DEI that are transparent and widely promulgated. These are often available from your institution's DEI officer and readily available through a wide range of professional organizations. Metrics should include explicit measures of faculty, staff, trainee, and student distribution and recruitment (especially by rank), resource allocation (e.g., compensation, space, staff support), and other indicators of DEI such as speaker invitations and recognition in publications, portraits, and photographs.

Your use of metrics should be accompanied by specific actions to address any biases that are detected (e.g., unconscious bias in search committee discussions) [29]. Additionally, you should perform periodic climate surveys of faculty, staff, trainees, and students as indicators of the effectiveness of your DEI programs, and use the results to institute changes and create new opportunities to continuously improve the experiences of all the members of your department.

References

1. Page SE. The diversity bonus: how great teams pay off in the knowledge economy. Princeton: Princeton University Press; 2017. ISBN 978-0691191539.
2. American Hospital Association. Health equity snapshot: a toolkit for action. https://www.aha.org/system/files/media/2020/12/ifdhe_snapshot_survey_FINAL.pdf. Accessed 19 Mar 2023.
3. Kelly T, Rodriguez SB. Expanding underrepresented in medicine to include lesbian, gay, bisexual, transgender, and queer individuals. Acad Med. 2022;97:1605–9. https://doi.org/10.1097/ACM.0000000000004720.
4. Plews-Ogan ML, Bell TD, Townsend G, Canterbury RJ, Wilkes DS. Acting wisely: eliminating negative bias in medical education – part 2: how can we do better? Acad Med. 2020;95:516–22. https://doi.org/10.1097/ACM.0000000000003700.
5. Roberts LW. Moving together toward health professions equity in academic medicine. Acad Med. 2022;97:1725–6. https://doi.org/10.1097/ACM.0000000000004989.
6. Ross PT, Lypson ML, Byington CL, Sanchez JP, Wong BM, Kumagai AK. Learning from the past and working in the present to create an antiracist future for academic medicine. Acad Med. 2020;95:1781–6. https://doi.org/10.1097/ACM.0000000000003756.

7. Conrad P, Carr P, Knight S, Renfrew MR, Dunn MB, Pololi L. Hierarchy as a barrier to advancement for women in academic medicine. J Womens Health. 2009;19:799–805. https://doi.org/10.1089/jwh.2009.1591.
8. Das D, Geynisman-Tan J, Mueller M, Kenton K. The leadership landscape: the role of gender in current leadership positions in obstetrics and gynecology departments. J Minim Invasive Gynecol. 2022;29:952–60. https://doi.org/10.1016/j.jmig.2022.03.013.
9. Hobgood CD, Draucker C. Barriers, challenges, and solutions: what can we learn about leadership in academic medicine from a qualitative study of emergency medicine women chairs? Acad Med. 2022;97:1656–64. https://doi.org/10.1097/ACM.0000000000004772.
10. Lipscomb MF, Bailey DN, Howell LP, Johnson R, Joste N, Leonard DGB, et al. Women in academic pathology: pathways to department chair. Acad Pathol. 2021;8:23742895211010322. https://doi.org/10.1177/23742895211010322.
11. Sethuraman KN, Lin M, Rounds K, Fang A, Lall M, Parsons M, et al. Here to chair: gender differences in the path to leadership. Acad Emerg Med. 2021;28:993–1000. https://doi.org/10.1111/acem.14221.
12. Thorndyke LE, Milner RJ, Jaffe LA. Endowed chairs and professorships: a new frontier in gender equity. Acad Med. 2022;97:1643–9. https://doi.org/10.1097/ACM.0000000000004722.
13. Vaidya NA. Women chairs in psychiatry: a collective reflection. Acad Psychiatry. 2006;30:315–8. https://doi.org/10.1176/appi.ap.30.4.315.
14. Odei BC, Jagsi R, Diaz DA, Addison D, Arnett A, Odei JB, et al. Evaluation of equitable racial and ethnic representation among departmental chairs in academic medicine, 1980-2019. JAMA Netw Open. 2021;4(5):e2110726. https://doi.org/10.1001/jamanetworkopen.2021.10726.
15. Xierali IM, Nivet MA, Rayburn WF. Diversity of department chairs in family medicine at US medical schools. J Am Board Fam Med. 2022;35:152–7. https://doi.org/10.3122/jabfm.2022.01.210298.
16. Yancy CW, Bauchner H. Diversity in medical schools: need for a new bold approach. JAMA. 2020;325:31–2. https://doi.org/10.1001/jama.2020.23601.
17. Yu PT, Parsa PV, Hassanein O, Rogers SO, Chang DC. Minorities struggle to advance in academic medicine: a 12-year review of diversity at the highest levels of America's teaching institutions. J Surg Res. 2013;182:212–8. https://doi.org/10.1016/j.jss.2012.06.049.
18. Morris DB, Gruppuso PA, McGee NA, Murillo AL, Grover A, Adashi EY. Diversity of the national medical student body – four decades of inequities. N Engl J Med. 2021;384:1661–8. https://doi.org/10.1056/NEJMsr2028487.
19. Greenwood BN, Carnahan S, Huang L. Patient-physician gender concordance and increased mortality among female heart attack patients. Proc Natl Acad Sci U S A. 2018;115:8569–74. https://doi.org/10.1073/pnas.1800097115.
20. Greenwood BN, Hardeman R, Huang L, Sojourner A. Physician-patient racial concordance and disparities in birthing mortality for newborns. Proc Natl Acad Sci. 2020;117:21194–200. https://doi.org/10.1073/pnas.1913405117.
21. Diaz T, Navarro JR, Chen EH. An institutional approach to fostering inclusion and addressing racial bias: implications for diversity in academic medicine. Teach Learn Med. 2020;32:110–6. https://doi.org/10.1080/10401334.2019.1670665.
22. Rosenkranz KM, Arora TK, Termuhlen PM, Stain SC, Misra S, Dent D, et al. Diversity, equity and inclusion in medicine: why it matters and how do we achieve it? J Surg Educ. 2021;78:1058–65. https://doi.org/10.1016/j.jsurg.2020.11.013.
23. Pino-Jones AD, Cervantes L, Flores S, Jones CD, Keach J, Ngov L-K, et al. Advancing diversity, equity, and inclusion in hospital medicine. J Hosp Med. 2021;16:198–203. https://doi.org/10.12788/jhm.3574.
24. Executive Leadership Program in Academic Medicine. https://drexel.edu/medicine/academics/womens-health-and-leadership/elam. Accessed 17 Mar 2022.
25. Carol Emmott Foundation. https://carolemmottfoundation.org/carol-emmott-fellowship/. Accessed 19 Mar 2023.

26. Center for Women in Academic Medicine and Science. https://cwams.org/category/faculty-network/. Accessed 19 Mar 2023.
27. Kamceva M, Kyerematen B, Spigner S, Bunting S, Li-Sauerwine S, Yee J, et al. More work, less reward: the minority tax on US medical students. J Wellness. 2022;4:5. https://doi.org/10.55504/2578-9333.1116.
28. Rodriguez JE, Campbell KM, Pololi LH. Addressing disparities in academic medicine: what of the minority tax? BMC Med Educ. 2015;15:1–5. https://doi.org/10.1186/s12909-015-0290-9.
29. Blair-Loy M, Mayorova OV, Cosman PC, Fraley SI. Can rubrics combat gender bias in faculty hiring? Science. 2022;377:35–7. https://doi.org/10.1126/science.abm2329.

Chapter 8
Building Collaborations and Collegiality

The Value Added

"What Are the Benefits of Promoting Faculty Collaboration and Collegiality?"

Faculty collaboration and collegiality go hand in hand, and together they promote success across all your department's missions. Nevertheless, some faculty are reluctant to collaborate because they fear losing control of their projects or having their ideas appropriated by collaborators. Some also are concerned about sharing recognition with others, especially at institutions where rewards and recognition (e.g., promotion, resources, bonuses) are limited to first/senior authors and principal investigators. Unfortunately, the importance and benefits of collaboration are usually not emphasized in curricula and often must be learned from practical experience during one's career [1]. Both collaboration and collegiality enhance the clinical care of patients, improve research, facilitate medical education and training, and enhance community service [2].

Collaboration among faculty usually creates synergies that can result in access to more resources through shared facilities and programs. Evidence of this is the establishment of centers and institutes, which by definition are interdisciplinary. Moreover, collaboration across widely diverse disciplines is often the basis for the greatest innovation. Collegiality is a key behavior that promotes and facilitates collaboration; reciprocally, creating collaborative programs can engender collegiality, which together improves morale, well-being, and productivity. Collaboration and collegiality also enhance understanding and respect across different disciplines, facilitate DEI, and create new research, clinical, educational, and community service opportunities. These can extend well beyond other medical school departments to departments in other schools in the health sciences (e.g., pharmacy, nursing,

F. Sanfilippo et al., *Lead, Inspire, Thrive*, https://doi.org/10.1007/978-3-031-41177-9_8

dentistry, public health) and university (e.g., business, law, social sciences), as well as throughout the health-care services programs.

Research and Clinical Faculty Relationships

"How Can I Encourage Collaboration Between Research and Clinical Faculty?"

Collaboration between clinical and research faculty is important for the success of your department. Nonclinical research faculty are often eager to have clinical collaborations to make their basic, translational, or health services research projects more clinically relevant and therefore attractive to more funding agencies. Likewise, clinical faculty, who are often overloaded with patient care responsibilities and may have less research experience and technical expertise, frequently seek collaboration on research projects relevant to their clinical interests that will strengthen their academic portfolios. Indeed, there usually are multiple opportunities for clinical faculty to be co-investigators on research grants and for research faculty to collaborate on clinical trials.

A useful way to stimulate discussion and potential collaboration among research and clinical faculty is through departmental retreats. Additional ways to stimulate such interactions include:

- Committees—appointing clinical and research faculty to appropriate department- and institution-wide committees.
- Courses—assigning research and clinical faculty to joint teaching activities, particularly with the movement toward curricular integration of basic and clinical sciences.
- Events—scheduling educational and social functions that include both research and clinical faculty.
- Fundraising—raising support for joint clinical research programs, faculty, students, and facilities.
- Retreats—including topics that engage both clinical and research faculty and programs.
- Seminars and symposia—including presentations by research and clinical faculty of their scholarly work.

Stimulating Collaboration

"What Are Appropriate Incentives to Stimulate Collaboration?"

There are several incentives you can provide to stimulate collaboration, especially across disciplines and between research and clinical faculty, along with the students and trainees they educate (e.g., PhD students and post-doctoral fellows, medical students, residents, and clinical fellows). A common incentive is creating a "seed grant" funding program to stimulate collaborative research projects between research and clinical faculty, as well as among faculty in different subspecialties in your department and even with faculty in other departments. Such projects may serve as pilot projects to support subsequent application for extramural grant support, which in turn can generate additional funds to sustain the seed grant program. You also might consider incorporating financial incentives for collaboration and collegiality into your faculty compensation plans (see Chap. 19, section "Incentives and Bonuses").

Whenever using departmental funds for a specific program, it is important to be transparent and engage faculty for their input and approval. You can include incentives for collaboration as part of your departmental strategic planning and budgeting processes by considering such expenses as an investment in faculty development as well as supporting your department's "R&D." You may also create a connection between "sources and uses" for funds generated by clinical and research faculty productivity (e.g., clinical revenue, cost recovery for grants) to support incentives that involve both clinical and research faculty.

Promoting Collegiality

"How Should I Promote Collegiality?"

Collegiality is a characteristic of personal behavior as well as a critical component of constructive organizational cultures (see Chap. 6, section "Understanding Culture Types and Styles"). In addition to facilitating collaboration, it enhances productive negotiation, teamwork, fundraising, and individual wellness. Although difficult to evaluate and somewhat controversial, a number of institutions consider collegiality an important characteristic for promotion, and some even identify it as the cultural attribute most responsible for success [3, 4].

There are several ways you can promote collegiality in your department. Clearly communicating its value, importance, and characteristics and providing expectations of collegial behavior are all valuable. Providing incentives, rewards, and recognition for collegiality can be useful but must be based on objective criteria and instituted carefully. Including collegiality and collaboration as factors in faculty, staff, trainee, and student recruitment can also enhance these behaviors in your department, as can establishing a "buddy" system to pair appropriate team members to help these new hires. That said, your personal example in engaging and dealing with others is probably the most important way to promote collegiality and collaboration in your department [5].

References

1. Gottlieb M, Grossman C, Rose E, Sanderman W, Akel F, Swaminathan A, et al. Academic primer series: five key papers about team collaboration relevant to emergency medicine. West J Emerg Med. 2017;18:303–10. https://doi.org/10.5811/westjem.2016.11.31212.
2. Lerner S, Magrane D, Friedman E. Teaching teamwork in medical education. Mt Sinai J Med. 2009;76:318–29. https://doi.org/10.1002/msj.20129.
3. American Association of University Professors: on collegiality as a criterion for faculty evaluation. 2016. https://aaup.org/report/collegiality-criterion-faculty-evaluation. Accessed 10 Oct 2022.
4. Koskenranta M, Kuivila H, Pramila-Savukoski S, Mannisto M, Mikkonen K. Development and testing of an instrument to measure the collegiality competence of social and health care educators. Nurse Educ Today. 2022;113:105388. https://doi.org/10.1016/j.nedt.2022.105388.
5. Kelly R. 7 ways a chair can promote collegiality. Academic Briefing. 2017. https://academic-briefing.com/human-resources/collegiality/promote-collegiality. Accessed 10 Oct 2022.

Chapter 9
Promoting Work-Life Balance

Developing a Successful Departmental Work-Life Balance

"How Can I Promote a Successful Work-Life Balance for Members of My Department?"

Just as it is important for you to develop your own personal work-life balance (see Chap. 36), it is important to recognize that the work-life balance of your faculty, staff, and students/trainees has a profound impact on their well-being and performance. There is considerable recent literature on changes in physician work hours and their implication for work-life balance [1–4]. There are important ways you can promote an appropriate and healthy work-life balance to enhance wellness for members of your department that are discussed in subsequent chapters on Career Development and Wellness for faculty (Chap. 18), students and trainees (Chap. 22), and staff (Chap. 25).

For most faculty, staff, trainees, and students, a healthy work-life balance is not easy to establish and will vary from individual to individual depending on their own personal circumstances. Because signals from their supervisors and the department play an important role in their approach, your messaging as leader on why and how to develop a successful work-life balance can have an enormous impact. There are several ways to send this message:

- Emphasizing the importance at departmental meetings.
- Explaining the benefits of personal time.
- Holding supervisors accountable for promoting a positive work-life balance.
- Making wellness and resilience programs easily accessible.
- Offering flexibility in work hours and remote work.
- Providing advice on how to proactively manage and balance time at work.
- Using departmental publications and newsletters.

F. Sanfilippo et al., *Lead, Inspire, Thrive*, https://doi.org/10.1007/978-3-031-41177-9_9

However, as a key role model in your department, the most important message you send is how you balance your own work-life activities.

Work Time

"How Can I Help Members of My Department Better Manage Their Administrative Work Time?"

The major issue in work-life balance is how to manage and allocate time for both work and personal time. For most members of your department, there is not enough time in the day to manage their workload and have enough additional time for their personal needs and interests. This is especially true for time spent by faculty on administrative functions that reduce their time for their academic and clinical activities, which exacerbates problems with work-life balance and wellness. Likewise, staff as well as students and trainees who must deal with inefficient processes or inadequate resources have less time to get their work done.

For clinical faculty, the administrative burden of time spent beyond direct patient contact in recording and documenting compliance requirements has escalated to the point where it has become one of the leading causes of burnout. Moreover, for women and under-represented groups, there is often a greater number of requests for mentoring and serving on committees that add to their administrative time burden as a "minority tax" (see Chap. 7).

There are many ways to help members of your department manage their administrative work time. Although it is tempting to ask the most productive members of your department to sit on committees and assist with administrative functions, you should be careful to balance the potential departmental benefit of their service with the added workload they would have to assume.

Probably the greatest help you can provide is from advice and the example you set for managing administrative time. Practical advice can be provided at meetings and through departmental communications and can include information and guidance on how best to appropriately use communication tools (e.g., e-mails, texts, calls) more efficiently and effectively (see Chap. 5), how to gain control of scheduling and calendars that includes scheduled free time blocked off to catch up on work, and how to deal with requests to attend meetings and sit on committees. Many of these approaches for saving time are detailed in Chap. 36, section "Time Management at Work."

An important message to send repeatedly, especially to the busiest and most productive members of your department, is that they shouldn't say yes to take on more work unless they can say no to something else they are doing.

"How Can I Help Members of My Department Better Manage Their Professional Work Time?"

Faculty, staff, students, and trainees all should be spending most of their work time on the primary responsibilities of their positions, whether clinical, research, educational, or administrative. Nevertheless, you may be able to provide advice about potential opportunities to save time and effort in each of these areas. In so doing, you should emphasize that long hours do not necessarily equal productive hours [5].

For faculty involved in clinical service, they may be able to better utilize assistance from mid-level providers by allowing them to practice at their full scope of training. Likewise, identifying and using appropriate decision support tools can save time, and working with those who schedule clinical appointments can also help to avoid over- or under-booking.

For faculty involved in research, it may be helpful to advise them to be more selective and focused on the impact of their efforts when considering collaborations and writing papers. Likewise, you can advise them to evaluate the potential cost-benefit of utilizing additional technical or administrative support to increase their productivity, but you should be prepared for requests to provide such resources.

For educational activities, advice on using online, virtual, and simulation technologies can potentially increase efficiency and effectiveness for both the instructor and learner; again, you should be ready for resource requests. Guidance for administrative staff similarly may be focused on identifying appropriate technology and assistance from staff to increase productivity and save time.

Personal Time

"How Can I Help Members of My Department Better Utilize and Appreciate the Importance of Personal Time?"

Ensuring appropriate personal time for members of your department is critical to their work-life balance, wellness, and ultimately their satisfaction and productivity at work. Although most faculty, staff, and students/trainees understand this, the demands of work, especially in an academic health-care setting, can often overwhelm the desire and need to take appropriate personal time. If personal time does not become an explicit priority that is scheduled, it often becomes sacrificed for work.

Your messaging, role modeling, and reinforcement of the importance of spending appropriate time for family, friends, and personal activities are critical in allowing members of your department to feel comfortable in taking time away from work. You should remind members of your department that family (including oneself) should come first, especially for those involved in caring for children, parents, or other family members, as well as for dealing with personal issues, especially involving their own health and well-being.

You also should demonstrate by your own actions and messaging that personal time for oneself is essential in order to stay refreshed, reduce stress, improve resilience, and avoid burnout. Show others that the enjoyment of life outside of work, including hobbies, sports, fun activities with family and friends, and simple rest and relaxation, is an essential part of everyday life. Significant personal time for vacations is also important for good work-life balance. Let members of your department know that they should feel that taking personal time away from work can benefit their physical and mental health, strengthen their social connection with family and friends, and increase their satisfaction and productivity.

References

1. Brown CVR, Joseph BA, Davis K, Jurkovich GJ. Modifiable factors to improve work-life balance for trauma surgeons. J Trauma Acute Care Surg. 2021;90:122–8. https://doi.org/10.1097/TA.0000000000002910.
2. Goldman AL, Barnett ML. Changes in physician work hours and implications for workforce capacity and work-life balance, 2001-2021. JAMA Intern Med. 2022;183:106. https://doi.org/10.1001/jamainternmed.2022.5792.
3. Hung DY, Mujal G, Jin A, Liang S-Y. Road to better work-life balance? Lean redesigns and daily work time among primary care physicians. J Gen Intern Med. 2022;37:2358–64. https://doi.org/10.1007/s11606-021-07178-6.
4. Tawfi DS, Shanafelt TD, Dyrbye LN, Sinsky CA, West CP, Davis AS, et al. Personal and professional factors associated with work-life integration among US physicians. JAMA Netw Open. 2021;4:e2111575. https://doi.org/10.1001/jamanetworkopen.2021.11575.
5. Bartlett MJ, Arslan FN, Bankston A, Sarabipour S. Ten simple rules to improve academic work-life balance. PLoS Comput Biol. 2021;17:e1009124. https://doi.org/10.1371/journal.pcbi.1009124.

Chapter 10
Negotiation

When to Negotiate

"When Should I Negotiate Rather Than Just Agree with a Proposal or Counter-Proposal?"

If you have been offered a proposal or counter-proposal, you should consider negotiating rather than just accepting the proposal or counter-proposal when you believe that:

- The terms being offered are not acceptable.
- The terms are not explicit or need clarification.
- The assumptions behind the proposal or counter-proposal are incorrect.
- Additional considerations could be included to create a better agreement.
- Greater total value could be created for all parties to the agreement.

"When Should I Start a New Negotiation in Response to a Proposal?"

Although it may be tempting to simply offer a new proposal or a counter-proposal to the one provided, it may be better to start a fresh negotiation when:

- You don't know the other side well.
- You do not know what the other side might value.
- You think that additional parties might become involved.

In the long run, starting a fresh negotiation may save time by avoiding multiple rounds of point-counterpoint.

© The Author(s), under exclusive license to Springer Nature
Switzerland AG 2023
F. Sanfilippo et al., *Lead, Inspire, Thrive*,
https://doi.org/10.1007/978-3-031-41177-9_10

How to Negotiate

"How Should I Negotiate for Departmental Resources Such as Budget, Space, Personnel, Etc.?"

As much as possible, provide quantitative data supporting the need for the resources you are requesting, e.g., salary surveys, space justification based on clinical service volume and research-grant funding, personnel needs based upon workload volume, and Graduate Medical Education (GME) funds for clinical teaching. Data do not lie, but there can be significant disagreements about how the data are interpreted.

As in any negotiation, it is important to understand what the other parties value and how they might benefit from the final agreement. So be sure to clearly and accurately quantify the net benefits (e.g., return on investment) to the institution(s) or units providing the resources. Also, emphasize the potential impact of any missed opportunities and anticipated problems if an agreement is not realized. Whenever possible, dry-run your proposal and potential negotiating options with trusted members of your leadership team.

If part or all of your request cannot be met, it usually is helpful to put yourself in the position of the decision-maker, simulating a situation in which you are not able to meet requests of your own faculty. Try to behave and understand as you would want your faculty to behave and understand if you were unable to meet their requests.

It is wise to suspend or end a negotiation when it becomes counter-productive. Be objective and not accusatory. Avoid confrontation and demands during a negotiation, and, above all, don't turn the discussion and negotiation into a personal conflict with your boss(es) or their surrogates. It is fine to agree to disagree in a collegial manner, but not worth ending a relationship over a negotiation for resources.

"How Should I Negotiate When Dealing with Faculty and Staff Requests for Resources, Promotion, Etc.?"

You should always be data-driven in evaluating a faculty and/or staff request. Ask for quantitative data supporting the request with appropriate reference points for justification. Also, ask for an objective assessment of the net benefits to the department and institution (e.g., return on investment over time), and explore the negative consequences of not being able to fulfill the request.

In negotiating with faculty or staff, it is often useful to include an intermediary who is trusted by you and the faculty or staff member. Avoid confrontation, don't engage in a personal conflict, and suspend or end the negotiation if it becomes counter-productive, bitter, or personal.

"How Should I Negotiate for Personal Issues Such as Salary, Space, Staff Support, Etc.?"

As above, be sure to have objective data to justify the request. Be transparent on the personal importance of the request and be explicit on how the response to the request may impact you and the department.

It may be helpful to discuss your proposal and potential negotiating options with trusted friends, family, and mentors beforehand, and, as appropriate, you may wish to engage your most trusted departmental leaders. Again, avoid confrontation or demands, and don't let the negotiation turn into a personal conflict.

"Do's and Don'ts"

As emphasized above, providing documentation and appropriate objective data is a necessary component of negotiation. However, perhaps the most important aspect of any successful negotiation is developing mutual trust among the parties and the understanding that all parties should be transparent throughout the process.

If parties cannot be trusted, documentation becomes even more important, but its validity and interpretation will likely be questioned. In such circumstances, a mutually trusted and objective third party may be necessary. Again, avoid confrontation, demands, and personal conflicts. Try to understand the perspective of the other parties in the negotiation and try to make the outcome an equitable "win-win" for all [1]. These factors are particularly important when dealing with such major issues as affiliations and mergers, especially if the parties have different cultures (e.g., academic versus non-academic).

Unfortunately, despite these principles, many view negotiations as an adversarial process that requires "hard positional bargaining." Instead, you always should consider principled negotiation as a process in which shared interests, mutually satisfying options, and fair standards are emphasized and can create benefits and value for all parties [2–5].

References

1. Weiss A-PC. Negotiation: how to be effective. J Hand Surg Am. 2017;42:53–6. https://doi.org/10.1016/j.jhsa.2016.10.009.
2. Castaneda P. The art of negotiation: avoiding positional bargaining and getting to yes. J Pediatr Orthopaedics. 2022;42:547–9. https://doi.org/10.1097/BPO.0000000000002059.
3. Eisenmann BS, Wagner RD, Reece EM. Practical negotiation for medical professionals. Semin Plastic Surg. 2018;32:166–71. https://doi.org/10.1055/s-0038-1672149.

4. Nguyen HB, Thomson C, Jarjour NN, Dixon AE, Liesching TN, Schnapp LN. Leading change and negotiation strategies for division leaders in clinical medicine. Chest. 2019;156:1246–53. https://doi.org/10.1016/j.chest.2019.06.019.
5. Sambuco D, Dabrowska A, Decastro R, Steward A, Ubel A, Jagsi R. Negotiation in academic medicine: narratives of faculty researchers and their mentors. Acad Med. 2013;88:505–11. https://doi.org/10.1097/ACM.0b013e318286072b.

Part III
Operational Issues

All good leaders know that in addition to the leadership skills needed to create a vision and set priorities, there are many management and administrative issues, especially involving personnel, space, and finances that must be constantly addressed to run a department successfully. How your department is organized and structured will impact its operations, culture, and performance. Developing an effective strategic plan and appropriate budgets is necessary to define the goals, tactics, resources, and metrics that address expectations and priorities across all the missions of your department. It is likewise important to balance and align your faculty activities and departmental programs in education, research, health care delivery, and public service appropriately. An even greater challenge is managing change, especially in dealing with occasional and unanticipated crises, whether financial, environmental, or personal. Developing the right team of faculty and staff, along with appropriate policies and practices, is critical for your success in managing these operational issues.

Chapter 11
Organizing the Department

Leadership Positions

"What Leadership Positions Should I Keep, Change, and Create?"

Your first priority in organizing your department must be getting the right people "on the bus." The best leaders surround themselves with people smarter in their areas of expertise than themselves; direct them to make decisions aligned with the culture, vision, and priorities of the department; and don't look over their shoulder. Of these departmental leaders, your senior administrator, executive deputy/vice chair, and "chief of staff" can be the most important [1].

Leadership positions to consider for your department may include vice/deputy chairs, division heads, program directors, administrative managers, and section directors, who can be assigned to oversee mission areas (e.g., clinical services, education, research, community outreach) and important activities such as DEI, information technology (IT), faculty development, and finance [2]. Each leadership position should serve a specific purpose in your organizational structure and be led by an individual having expertise and a strong interest in that function. In some cases, it also may be useful to create a position primarily to utilize the talents of a superior individual, or to provide additional titles/positions with reasonable cost, time, effort, and authority as a means of recognition or reward.

The most effective teams have members who bring diverse experiences, expertise, and perspectives to the group (see Chap. 7). It is important that the team has members with the skills necessary to lead in the current environment and members with the ability to envision and guide the changes needed to succeed in the future.

Several factors should influence your decision to keep, change, or create a leadership position, and retain, remove, or appoint a leader. For leadership positions, you should consider how well the position aligns with the department's strategic

© The Author(s), under exclusive license to Springer Nature Switzerland AG 2023

F. Sanfilippo et al., *Lead, Inspire, Thrive*,
https://doi.org/10.1007/978-3-031-41177-9_11

priorities and operational structure, and what resources are available to support the position. Similarly, for the leaders in these positions, you should consider how much the individual supports the department's strategic priorities, values, and your vision for the department, how well you know and trust the individual, and how much the faculty, staff, and institution support the individual.

Department size, complexity, operations, and missions also should be considered when you are appointing leaders, and appropriate input from stakeholders within and outside the department should be solicited. The roles, responsibilities, authority, accountability, and reporting relationships should be carefully defined for each position and clearly agreed upon with the appointed leader.

As mentioned previously (see Chap. 5), many faculty, staff, students, and trainees may be hesitant to bring issues to you directly, so it is important to have individuals who are trustworthy and approachable in your leadership positions. Creating a formal or informal "chief of staff" position filled by a senior staff or faculty member who is highly trusted by members of your department can be of great help in receiving and transmitting difficult messages. Similarly, since your personal EA is the usual point of contact for reaching you, that person should be someone well trusted by members of your department and especially other institutional leaders, as well as by your personal contacts and family members. Your EA should be an individual you trust to handle the most delicate of messages and issues, who gets to know your habits well, and someone in whom you have confidence to make the right decisions about your priorities for scheduling meetings and events.

One of the biggest mistakes and regrets of good leaders is not removing problem lieutenants soon enough. When faced with removing non- or counter-productive leaders, always proceed carefully. Get internal and external support; watch for "end-arounds" and push-back that they may instigate with institutional leaders or external stakeholders, especially if they have been in the position a long time, have high visibility, or receive substantial compensation. If significant culture or performance change is needed in the department, using leadership positions to kill "sacred cows" as well as to create "disciples" and "apostles" can be very effective.

Building Your Team

"Should I Create a Departmental Leadership Team (e.g., 'Executive Committee'), and, If So, What Should Be Its Composition and Its Role?"

A powerful and essential asset in running your department is your leadership team. Outstanding teams can greatly expand the scope, scale, and performance of you and your department. An often-used metaphor for department leaders is that they are like the conductor of an orchestra, with the resulting symphony being dependent on how well each player performs individually *and* together. Similarly, the success of a manager or coach of a sports team is highly dependent on how they position their players and motivate them to play as a team for a common goal of achieving expectations [3].

Outstanding teams are diverse in background, experience, and viewpoints; they provide input from several perspectives and are highly innovative [3, 4]. You should create your small "Executive Committee" leadership team from the best of these leaders and avoid making important decisions without getting their input and advice. Good Executive Team members are strong team leaders and team players who are more committed to the overall success of the department than just their unit or themselves.

To create an efficient and effective executive leadership team, you should try to have the smallest number of highly engaged individuals that provide the broadest diversity of input and oversight (i.e., a tightly knit, diverse group of experts committed to the success of the department). An Executive Committee that attempts to represent all sections of the department can become too unwieldy. Furthermore, section representatives may feel that it is their job to protect their unit's turf, rather than focusing on the department's overall interests and welfare. Unless stated otherwise, members of your executive team should keep all discussion and decisions strictly confidential.

To derive the most benefit from the advice of your Executive Committee, and to keep them engaged, you should have regular standing meetings (usually weekly) with a standard agenda that can include review, discussion, and input/approval on items such as:

- Activities, problems, and opportunities involving departmental programs and sections.
- Departmental proposals and issues, prior to bringing them to the full department.
- Faculty/staff/student/trainee performance, recruitments, and retentions.
- Institutional issues and initiatives.
- Progress on departmental initiatives, goals, strategy.
- Setting the agenda for faculty/departmental meetings, retreats, events, etc.

"How Should I Delegate Authority to My Faculty and Administrative Leaders?"

All leaders should have their authority aligned with their responsibilities and accountability. Providing a leader with responsibility but not authority is inappropriate if you expect to hold them accountable, and often will lead to unnecessary conflicts and problems. You should determine how much authority you wish to grant to each leader and provide the appropriate responsibility and accountability.

It often is best to provide less responsibility and authority at first, especially if someone is in a new role, and grant them more over time as is suitable, since it is generally harder to delegate substantial authority/responsibility to a leader and subsequently pull back. Delegating the most authority and responsibility to those who are most trustworthy and committed to the overall success of the department also sends a positive message about the importance of teamwork.

The relationship between your lieutenants and other department members must be based upon mutual trust and recognition of their importance, but acknowledgement that ultimate accountability and responsibility rests with you [5]. For high-functioning leaders, you should delegate to them decisions *within* the divisions, programs, and units that they oversee. For issues *between* divisions, programs, and units, you should delegate decisions to the appropriate leaders of those units working together as a group. All delegated decisions should be communicated to you and your Executive Committee so you are all aware of them in case issues or questions should arise. Likewise, all disagreements between unit leaders should be brought to you and your Executive Committee for discussion and resolution.

You should not micromanage the work of your leaders or their teams. Micromanagement is an indication that you believe your lieutenants are not able to meet responsibilities, or that you are incapable of delegating authority. If the problem is that they are not accomplishing assigned tasks with appropriate time and resources, they should be counseled and replaced if they subsequently are unable to meet expectations. If you have trust and confidence in your leadership team members' commitment and abilities, you should not interfere with their work, and provide help and advice only when asked or needed.

A mistake of some leaders is to provide responsibility but usurp authority by micromanaging the way they do their job. There is a learning curve for everyone in a new leadership role, and you should handle new lieutenants the way you want your own supervisors to not micromanage how you do your job. Remember that well-intentioned advice to a lieutenant on how to do a job may be perceived much more like an expectation or command than just an idea or suggestion. Delegating appropriate responsibility and decision-making is an important sign of your trust in your team. Likewise, showing strong support rather than blame for team members who show initiative and make well-intentioned, well-informed mistakes that are aligned with department values, goals, and priorities is essential to have your team be innovative and opportunistic rather than too risk avoidant.

"How Should I Interact with My Faculty and Administrative Leaders?"

As appropriate, you should develop personal as well as professional relationships with your key leaders. Help them in their career development with advice and support, and consider them for awards and nominations to prestigious societies or other visible positions. You also should monitor their workload and that of their teams; when beyond reasonable expectations you should remind them of the need for appropriate work-life balance (see Chap. 9, section "Developing a Successful

Departmental Work-Life Balance), provide direction on priorities, and consider other internal or external resources to offer help (see Chap. 34).

It also can be helpful to explain your coaching style to your department faculty and staff, which may include descriptions of your methods for:

- Providing advice and assistance.
- Evaluating roles, responsibilities, and workload.
- Delegating authority and decision-making.
- Setting overall strategy, goals, and priorities.
- Celebrating and allocating rewards and recognition for successes.
- Providing support and encouragement for mistakes and failures.

Reciprocally, it is important to get feedback and input from your department about your performance, behavior, and interactions. Most individuals are hesitant about providing their boss with what may be perceived as criticism, so it is necessary to establish a high degree of trust and confidence among your faculty and staff leaders, and that you truly appreciate their candid and constructive advice on how you can improve. A good way to facilitate this is by asking specific questions about your potential areas of weakness and showing gratitude for their feedback.

In working with your lieutenants, you also should remember to respect the chain of command by not allowing subordinates to access you directly without having first gone through the leadership structure immediately above them. Allowing individuals to "jump over" their superiors will undermine those leaders. Obviously, there may be exceptions to this, especially if the superior is the problem.

Divisions and Sections

"What Are Successful Departmental Organizational Models?"

The best departmental organizational model is one that optimally serves the department, its strategic priorities, and its mission. It should be responsive to the nature and culture of the department; facilitate the productivity of your faculty, staff, students, and trainees; and help you provide the leadership needed to achieve the expectations of the institution. A department's organization often reflects tradition and accommodation of specific faculty and staff interests over time rather than what best serves its performance. A new chair can break the mold and create a new model, which is often easier for a leader from the outside to accomplish.

Successful departmental models can be structured in many ways, such as by missions (e.g., health care, research, education, outreach), services, academic programs, topics that span all missions, or a combination thereof. Regardless of structure, you should utilize key committees to ensure that there are good lines of communication and clear expectations about responsibilities across structural units, with each committee having a clearly defined charge [6].

"Should I Restructure the Department?"

If you are considering a restructure of your department, it is important to get input beforehand from internal and external stakeholders on how well or poorly they think the existing structure is working, and determine if the structure is in synchrony with the functions of the department. Upon refreshing an existing strategic plan or implementing a new one (see Chap. 12), you should assess how well the structure supports the new strategic goals and priorities. Determine if the departmental units complement and synergize each other across missions and subspecialties, or whether they compete. Also consider if there are parent or affiliated institutions (e.g., university, school, hospital, health system) that desire separate organizational structures for their activities. Study organizational models of peer departments at other institutions, as well as other departments at your institution. One department that underwent extensive reorganization and culture change experience was able to document rapid and sustained improvement in performance across missions [7].

Experts in organizational sciences (check with your business school) can be very helpful in assessing your current model and advising on changes. Test your potential departmental model by creating scenarios of "what if's" to determine how decision-making will flow. Have your organizational chart reviewed by department faculty (plan a retreat) and by school and other institutional leaders so that everyone understands the model and its rationale.

Operations and Administration

"How Should I Organize Administrative Staff to Best Support the Activities of the Department?"

The administrative organization of your department should reflect its size, complexity, and the parent organization(s) that are involved. Consolidating similar administrative functions (e.g., finance, operations) into shared-service models across departmental units may allow staffing for these activities with a higher level of expertise and less redundancy. Consider sharing staff with other departments, especially if you lead a small department. Ensure that reporting relationships are explicit and transparent, especially for activities that span institutions (e.g., hospital, medical school, other schools in the health sciences and university).

"How Do I Align Departmental Administrators and Staff Who Report to Different Parent Organizations (e.g., Hospital, University Campus)?"

The first step in aligning departmental administrative and operational staff who report outside the department is to evaluate the level of authority (control) exerted by the parent organization(s) over their activity and compensation, and then try to develop a mutually agreeable approach to managing them. These situations may include:

- Full control of personnel, operations, and budget by your department with accountability to the parent institution(s).
- Control of personnel and operations by the department with budget control by the parent institution(s).
- Control of personnel and operations by the parent institution(s) with budget allocated to the department.
- Control of institutional personnel (e.g., development, tech transfer, marketing, IT) by the department with joint funding and deemed status by the parent institution(s).
- Control of institutional personnel by the parent institution(s) with joint funding by the department.

In scenarios with differences among control of personnel, operations, and budget, there likely will be disparities in program responsibility and authority, making accountability ambiguous if not impossible. In such cases it is critically important for you to have a clear understanding with your parent organization(s) that their expectations of performance must be tempered by your lack of authority in one (or more) of these components. It is also important to attempt resolution of these issues by negotiation with the appropriate institutional leaders (see Chap. 10). In many cases, the parent organization(s) can provide you and your department with delegated authority or deemed status to fully manage the personnel, operations, and budget.

Meetings and Events

"How Should I Schedule and Utilize Departmental Meetings?"

One of the major issues impacting faculty and staff productivity is the time spent at meetings. These can vary from ad hoc meetings scheduled with specific participants to discuss or negotiate issues and opportunities, to standing department-wide meetings, such as grand rounds or faculty meetings to discuss strategic priorities and program activities. In any case, meetings take faculty and staff away from their normal activities and should be used judiciously.

As discussed above, scheduling regular (usually weekly) meetings with your leadership "Executive Committee" is important to ensure that issues are discussed and vetted on a regular basis, allowing you to get valuable input and your faculty and staff to be confident that they have members engaged in decision-making. Similarly, it is important to have regular (usually monthly or quarterly) "faculty" meetings to review progress and provide updates on activities, as well as regular (usually weekly) department-wide meetings (e.g., grand rounds, research seminars) to present mission-based activities by members of the department and invited guest speakers. Most departments also have a wide range of recurrent meetings that involve committee activities as well as mission and discipline-based programs that involve faculty, staff, and in many cases students and trainees.

There are several questions you should make sure that members of your department can answer before they schedule meetings:

- Why have the meeting?
- What is the agenda?
- Who really needs to attend?
- Can it be virtual or in-person?
- How long does it need to be?

The purpose and a written agenda for the meeting should be provided to invited participants beforehand so they can make an informed decision about attending and be prepared if they go. Moreover, participants at regularly scheduled meetings should be asked for their feedback on the value of the meeting and if the frequency, length, and venue (virtual or in-person) are appropriate.

"What Events Should I Consider Scheduling for the Department?"

Events are important opportunities for social engagement, and, in addition to the faculty and grand rounds meetings mentioned above, you should consider scheduling occasional departmental meetings that are primarily social events to bring department members together. These can include holiday events at the end of the calendar year (e.g., celebration of the year's activities), faculty/staff recognition events (for promotions, awards), and student/trainee recognition events at the end of the academic year (for degree awards, completion of training). Having any of these off-site at a social venue (club, restaurant) adds expense, but makes it "special" in a way that can promote collegiality and connection within the department.

"What Meetings Should I Consider Attending Personally?"

Of course, you should plan to attend all your Executive Committee and faculty meetings and as many department-wide meetings and special events as possible. If you have occasional conflicts for your standing Executive Committee, keep it scheduled and have your most senior deputy (e.g., executive vice chair) run the meeting. For other departmental meetings that you are asked to attend, follow your rule of seeing the purpose and agenda before deciding whether to attend. Likewise, for personal meetings requested by faculty or staff members, be sure to know the purpose and agenda beforehand. If not forthcoming, cancel the meeting, even at the last minute. This will reinforce your message to the department that meetings should be justified by forethought with an explicit agenda.

"How Should I Participate in Meetings?"

As discussed in Chap. 5, your speaking style, body language, and manner of presenting content and information can have a significant impact on others. Your communication and behavior at meetings will be observed closely by many and serve as a role model for some. Be sure to be clear and transparent when chairing a meeting and focus on being interactive rather than domineering when attending a meeting led by others. Remember that some members of your department may feel intimidated or inhibited when you are present at a meeting, especially if you are leading it, so try hard to be engaging. Meetings are great venues for you to demonstrate humility and humor. Solicit feedback from trusted participants on how to improve your effectiveness when leading a meeting as well as your behavior as a meeting participant.

References

1. Ness RB, Samet JM. How to be a department chair of epidemiology: a survival guide. Am J Epidemiol. 2010;172:747–51. https://doi.org/10.1093/aje/kwq268.
2. Dunnick NR. Leading an academic radiology department: using vice chairs. J Am Coll Radiol. 2015;12:1298–300. https://doi.org/10.1016/j.jacr.2015.05.013.
3. LaFasto F, Larson C. When teams work best: 6,000 team members and leaders tell what it takes to succeed. London: Sage Publications; 2001. ISBN 978-0761923664.
4. Lencioni PM. The five dysfunctions of a team: a leadership fable. San Francisco: Jossey-Bass; 2002. ISBN 978-0787960859.
5. Willett CG. Reflections from a chair: leadership of a clinical department at an academic medical center. Cancer. 2015;22:3795–8. https://doi.org/10.1002/cncr.29588.
6. Winstead DK. Advice for chairs of academic departments of psychiatry: the "ten commandments". Acad Psychiatr. 2006;30:298–300. https://doi.org/10.1176/appi.ap.30.4.298.

7. Sanfilippo F, Burns KH, Borowitz ML, Jackson JB, Hruban RH. The Johns Hopkins Department of Pathology novel organizational model: a 25-year ongoing experiment. Acad Pathol. 2018;5:2374289518811145. https://doi.org/10.1177/2374289518811145.

Chapter 12
Strategic Planning

Evaluating Your Departmental Strategic Plan

"What Is the Best Approach for Reviewing My Department's Current Strategic Plan?"

Presumably your department has an existing strategic plan. The strategic plan should outline your department's goals and therefore the use of resources, especially the time and effort of your faculty and staff, as well as space and funding. If you are a new chair, reviewing the existing plan should be one of your highest priorities, even if you were a member of the department and participated in the development of the existing plan. As a new department leader, it is important to ensure that resource allocation is in line with the expectations and priorities set with your appointment.

Strategic planning is a leadership function [1], and the first step in reviewing your department's current plan is to engage your faculty, staff, and other institutional stakeholders to determine:

- Their level of satisfaction with the current plan.
- How well it fits with expectations (see Chap. 3).
- If the assumptions used are still accurate.
- If the culture, resources, and environment have changed substantially.
- If the metrics being used for measuring performance are still appropriate.

With this information, the next step is to determine the magnitude of potential changes needed for the plan to meet your department's performance expectations. If only minor changes are needed, an update or "refresh" of the plan should be sufficient, but if significant changes are necessary, you should initiate a new strategic planning process (see below).

© The Author(s), under exclusive license to Springer Nature
Switzerland AG 2023
F. Sanfilippo et al., *Lead, Inspire, Thrive*,
https://doi.org/10.1007/978-3-031-41177-9_12

"What If I Think the Current Departmental Plan Needs to Be Revised or Completely Redone?"

First you should carefully and objectively document the inadequacies and problems you see from your review of the existing plan, especially as they relate to expectations set for the department. This documentation then should be shared and discussed with the faculty and key staff as well as with the institution leaders that provided the expectations leading to the current plan. Remember that it may take as much time, effort, and resources to revise an existing plan as it would to create a new one.

If you feel strongly that the current plan is inadequate, it is important to get a sense of the commitment and support of the faculty and staff to the existing plan that they created, as well as their potential resistance or anxiety in your attempt to change it or begin a new strategic planning process. If you are a new leader from the same department, some may wonder why you didn't object or raise issues when the existing plan was developed. If you came from another institution, some may feel you need more experience in the department to justify changing their current strategic plan.

You also should have a candid discussion with institutional leaders, peers, and other stakeholders about your sense of the plan's inadequacies and how strongly they think a new plan is needed. Their view on the willingness of your faculty and staff to initiate another planning process should be a very important factor in deciding how to proceed.

If after an appropriate review, both departmental and institutional leaders feel the existing plan is adequate, or they clearly do not support the development of a new plan, you should express your concerns simply and concisely with the potential consequences and missed opportunities of continuing with the current plan. However, you should willingly and graciously accept the reality that changing the plan at that time likely would be counter-productive. Nevertheless, it is important to identify and get agreement on the metrics you feel would justify a subsequent reassessment of the existing plan, and track them accordingly.

Refreshing an Existing Strategic Plan

"What If I Am Expected to Implement the Current Departmental Plan But Believe That It Is Inadequate?"

If a departmental strategic plan was developed prior to your recruitment with the understanding that you would simply implement that new plan, it would be very difficult to try to develop a new strategic plan because:

- It would suggest those involved in the plan were not competent.

- It would appear that you were reneging on an understanding and are unreliable.
- There probably would be strategic planning "fatigue" by faculty and staff.
- Resources for a new planning process would have to be prioritized over other needs.

If upon a more detailed review you feel the strategic plan is inadequate (see above), but there is an expectation for you to execute the existing plan, or if there is strong resistance to starting a new plan, you can consider an alternative process to update or "refresh" the existing plan.

There are important considerations in planning to "refresh" an existing strategic plan:

- Make it clear that you are not creating a new plan.
- Focus on expectations, assumptions, and priorities.
- Put a short timeframe (1–2 months) for the entire process.
- Engage a limited number of departmental leaders.
- Keep resource use (especially faculty time and effort) to a minimum.
- Use local assistance (e.g., HR) and consider bringing in peer consultants.
- Get departmental and institutional leadership endorsement for any significant changes in expectations, priorities, and resource allocation.
- Be transparent and communicate succinctly about the process and results.

Developing a New Strategic Plan

"When Should I Launch a New Departmental Strategic Planning Process?"

A new strategic planning process should be initiated if:

- There is no existing plan or the current plan is over 5 years old.
- The current plan is agreed to be inadequate based on expectations, assumptions, and priorities (see above).
- The external environment has changed significantly (e.g., new threats or opportunities).
- There is an expectation by institutional leadership that a new plan is needed.
- There are sufficient faculty and staff support, time, effort, and resources available.

"What If I Am Expected to Lead the Development and Implementation of a New Plan But Find Substantial Departmental Resistance?"

If you find little departmental support or significant resistance to developing a new plan, but an expectation from institutional leadership to do it, you should proceed cautiously. Remind the department that you have an institutional role and responsibilities and get an outside, independent review of the plan from peers or professionals to help evaluate the current plan. This will message that you are sensitive and responding to their concerns and help members of the department see the potential need for a new plan. Using the approach of "refreshing" the existing plan (see above) can also mitigate some resistance to developing a new plan and still allow for a review of issues, opportunities, and assumptions to develop new expectations and priorities for the department.

"How Should I Develop and Implement a New Strategic Plan?"

As leader, you have to be the visible director of your department's strategic planning and take ownership of the process, outcome, and implementation. However, the most important part of developing a strategic plan is actively engaging departmental, institutional, and other stakeholders so that they have a true feeling of ownership in the process and its results. Strategic plans may be more important for how they engage stakeholders rather than what they produce. Moreover, repetition of the themes and language of strategic planning in formal and informal discussions can have a significant effect on the culture of the department [2].

As the initiator and leader of the process, you should become familiar with the substantial literature on how to develop a strategic plan. Start by reviewing and updating the departmental mission statement along with the expected values that define departmental organizational culture and behavioral norms. These should resonate across the department as well as the institution and other stakeholders (e.g., alumni, donors, those being served by the department). If faculty and staff are highly engaged, this often will become a lengthy process with substantial debate about wordsmithing the mission and values. If successful, this phase should increase the level of commitment and engagement by faculty and staff and make the more objective aspects of the planning process easier and less contentious.

The ultimate goal and a key point of a strategic plan is the vision statement, i.e., how the department aspires to perform in the future with typically a 5-year target. The vision statement is made in the context of the mission, values, and environment of the department which together are the basis by which the strategic priorities are identified.

A common failing of strategic plans is listing too many strategic priorities. In most cases, only a few (less than 5) strategic priorities should be identified, which in turn are used to identify specific goals and the appropriate tactics to achieve them. The tactics in turn should determine how resources are allocated, especially involving budget, space, and dollars, as well as the efforts of faculty and staff. Common mistakes in strategic planning include not involving the right people, not addressing the most relevant issues because they are perceived as too burdensome or complex, and not linking the plan to the resources required for implementation [3].

A good approach to assess the environment for your strategic plan is to perform a SWOT (strengths, weaknesses, opportunities, and threats) analysis early in your tenure as leader (see Chap. 2). This will provide important information to guide the development of assumptions, priorities, goals, and a vision statement. One useful approach to strategic planning has been described by the Department of Medicine at the University of Toronto Faculty of Medicine [4].

Finally, it is critically important to identify the metrics that will be used to measure the success of the plan and the timing of assessments, which should be at least yearly. If something is not being measured, it is usually considered to not be important.

Some additional advice in preparing your strategic plan:

- Ensure that the plan is in alignment with the overall institutional master plan.
- Ensure that the strategic priorities and their timing are appropriate to your mission, values, and vision and realistic to your environment and potential resources.
- Include a timeframe (e.g., 5 years) that is tied to priorities and the vision statement.
- Require annual progress reports with outcome measures.
- Consider engaging an outside facilitator/consultant to provide expertise about the process, an objective viewpoint of how the plan is developing, and assistance to departmental staff.
- Assign a leader to each strategic priority of the plan and hold them accountable for advancing their component of the plan.
- Ensure that resource allocation and your budget process are consistent with the priorities identified in the plan.

Managing Change

"What Should I Know About Managing Change?"

By definition, creating a vision for the future with specific goals and expectations as part of a strategic plan will require changes to achieve it. Even a vision to stay in place for a high-performing organization will likely require adjustments in order to adapt to the internal and external changes that will naturally occur over time. Indeed, academic medicine is challenged by many rapid changes in all of its mission areas. Changing reimbursement policies; increasing awareness of health disparities, AI-based decision support, and virtual delivery models in health care; new methodologies, technology, questions, and approaches in research; innovative pedagogy and digital methodologies in education; and increasing attention to the social mission of medical schools will require unprecedented change and inevitably cause disruption in most medical school departments. Inspirational leadership, strategic vision, diverse perspectives, openness to new approaches, evidence-based evaluation, and more will be required for success in a continuously learning organization.

Resistance to change is a natural response (inertia is a powerful force!), so managing change can be challenging. This is especially true when a chair is new and from the outside, when the department feels satisfied with the status quo, or when there is a significant change in institutional leadership, priorities, and expectations. In some cases, driving incremental change can be as hard or harder than transformational change. In fact, changes normally become more anticipated and accepted during a crisis (see Chap. 16). The challenges and approaches in changing culture are addressed further in Chap. 6, section "Driving Culture Change".

"How Can I Manage the Changes Needed in My Department?"

There is substantial literature with numerous books, papers, and even a *Journal of Change Management* (https://www.tandfonline.com/journals/rjcm20) on managing change in a wide variety of situations using several different methods (e.g., Lewin 3-step, McKinsey 7-step, Kotter 8-step, Nudge Theory, etc.) [5]. However, in considering which approach and process to use, it is important first to determine what actually needs to be changed (e.g., behavior, culture, operations, organizational structure, staffing, processes, goals), why the change is needed (e.g., funding, space, personnel issues; new institutional leadership, priorities, expectations; internal, external crisis), the desired impact and timing of the change, the anticipated magnitude of resistance and support for the intended change, and your personal and departmental capacity to manage the change.

In addition to the extensive published and online resources available to help you and your team tailor a change management process to your specific needs, your institutional HR department may have resources that can help. Always seek advice from others who have dealt with similar issues, and consider using consultants in more complex situations or when your capacity or expertise for managing change is limited (see Chap. 34). Likewise, there are numerous executive education courses offered by business schools and companies that can help you personally become more adept about leading change management initiatives (see Chap. 33, section "Leadership Training"). Remember, your active engagement as leader is critical for managing any significant change successfully.

References

1. Brophy PD, Stevenson K, Kaczorowski J, Schriefer J. A proposed technique to enhance strategic plan implementation using continuous quality improvement methodologies. J Pediatr. 2020;224:1–9. https://doi.org/10.1016/j.jpeds.2020.01.060.
2. Mallon WT. Does strategic planning matter? Acad Med. 2019;94:1408–11. https://doi.org/10.1097/ACM.0000000000002848.
3. Rodriguez PFP, Peiro M. Strategic planning in healthcare organizations. Rev Esp Cardio. 2012;65:749–54. https://doi.org/10.1016/j.recesp.2012.04.005. (Spanish).
4. Levinson W, Axler H. Strategic planning in a complex academic environment: lessons from one academic health center. Acad Med. 2007;82:806–11. https://doi.org/10.1097/ACM.0b013e3180d08d14.
5. Phillips J, Klein JD. Change management: from theory to practice. TechTrends. 2023;67:189–97. https://doi.org/10.1007/s11528-022-00775-0.

Chapter 13
Resources

Resource Management

"How Should I Prioritize Allocation of My Limited Departmental Resources (People, Space, Funding) to Meet the Substantial Demands?"

People are your most important (and usually most expensive) asset and must be considered first when managing all your resources. The priorities of your departmental strategic plan are most directly linked to the faculty and staff needed for its implementation. In turn, appropriate space and equipment are needed to facilitate the activity of these personnel, all of which require funding.

To properly execute a strategic plan and meet expectations, it is critical that resources are prioritized in alignment with your strategic priorities and associated tactics. In simple terms, a formal or informal "cost-benefit" analysis that is linked to "sources and uses" is needed when you are considering the allocation of departmental resources. This is especially important when dealing with resources that may be provided from different parent institutions (e.g., hospital, university), affiliates, or external organizations (e.g., state, foundation).

© The Author(s), under exclusive license to Springer Nature
Switzerland AG 2023
F. Sanfilippo et al., *Lead, Inspire, Thrive*,
https://doi.org/10.1007/978-3-031-41177-9_13

People

"With So Many Departmental Needs and Opportunities, How Should I Prioritize Recruitment and Retention of Faculty and Staff?"

Faculty recruitment and retention should be tied to programmatic strategic priorities, especially if an individual will leverage and enhance the overall performance and productivity of other faculty in your department. Similarly, recruitment/retention of administrative staff should be based on the operational needs of the department, which can change significantly with the development of new technology and equipment that can streamline work and increase efficiency, as well as with quantitative or qualitative changes in activity, which can shift staff support needed for research, clinical, or educational activities.

It is advantageous to consider how a particular faculty member may span and increase collaboration across missions, disciplines, and specialties in your department, as well as other departments, centers, and programs across the university and health system (see below). In some cases, a productive senior faculty member may have a significant impact on the recruitment/retention of other faculty, as well as students and trainees who wish to work in their research or clinical program. Depending on your department's structure and when appropriate, the recruitment/retention of a faculty member should be made across departmental divisions/units/programs to add greater value and potential opportunities to the individual and department.

From the perspective of departmental goals and expectations, a careful analysis should be made of the opportunity costs of any recruitment/retention package, as well as the anticipated impact on your department's strategic priorities. From a financial standpoint, the effect of ongoing direct and indirect expenses on the financial status of the department should be assessed, especially considering annual margins and reserves (see Chap. 14). The timeframe of potential return should be realistic as it can vary dramatically, for example, from the time needed for junior faculty involved in basic research to obtain funding to fully cover expenses, to the time needed for new clinical faculty and staff involved in billing to substantially increase collections and net revenue.

"When Should I Consider Joint Recruitment or Retention of Faculty or Staff with Another Department or Center?"

You should consider joint recruitment and retention of faculty and staff with other departments and centers in the medical school and across your AHC/AMC and university, especially when your resources (e.g., funding, space, equipment) are limited or when an added synergy and opportunity for the individual can be created by sharing their expertise (see Chap. 11, section "Operations and Administration" and Chap. 17). In addition to the benefits of sharing resources with another department, requests for institutional resources to help recruit/retain faculty or staff are much more effective when coming from multiple department/school/center leaders (see Chap. 29). Likewise, it is often more attractive to the individual when their recruitment/retention comes from more than one department/center at an institution. For clinical faculty involved in teaching residents, you also should determine the potential for obtaining appropriate support from the institution that receives GME funding. Of course, you should expect that the department chair/center/institute director of jointly funded faculty or staff will assume that those individuals will be appropriately devoted to their department, center, or institute.

Jointly appointed faculty and staff must have a clearly delineated description of their role in both departments. Although one department is usually designated as the "home" department for administrative purposes, the compensation, bonuses, and merit promotions of jointly appointed faculty and staff members will normally require all involved departments/centers to participate. This can become complicated if there are disagreements, but is usually beneficial since it can increase flexibility and available resources.

"How Should I Allocate Resources to Support Faculty?"

Resources (e.g., staff support, space, equipment, etc.) should be prioritized to facilitate faculty working on programs that highly support the mission and strategic priorities of the department. Unfortunately, it is often difficult to determine if it is more appropriate to add support to high-performing faculty or those who might become high performers with additional support. The practical issue of which investment of resources eventually will generate additional resources also should be a consideration. You should always engage your leadership team for their evaluation and recommendations for faculty support (see Chap. 11, section "Building Your Team").

Whenever possible, try to centralize resources that support faculty into core units, especially for shared space and equipment, and staff support. This generally is more economical and efficient, especially when shared services/resources are across departments/centers, and may promote collaboration among faculty sharing equipment, space, or staff (see Chap. 8) [1]. Reciprocally, it also can create synergy among staff who provide the same type of support. Cross-coverage among these individuals can help maintain faculty support when staffing is constrained.

Space

"Is the Current Space Allocation in My Department Appropriate?"

Space is a precious resource with limited availability. A department can often generate money to purchase equipment and hire faculty, but sometimes space is not available at any cost. A common mistake on the part of new leaders is to assume that if they can find funding for a new program or equipment, the institution will provide space. Too often this expectation leads to disappointing outcomes for both the department and the institution, as well as for any donors that might have provided the support.

Space also is a valuable resource that can be used to generate funding, and is critical to facilitate productivity of faculty and staff across mission areas (hence the term "facilities"). There are many different ways in which institutions handle space allocation to departments, such as by linking research space to indirect cost recovery from grant funding, tying clinic space to patient and payer mix, and considering space required for staffing. As chair, you should make sure that you understand your institution's policies and practices regarding assignment of space.

As with other resources, your allocation of the department's space for faculty activities should be based on productivity and strategic priorities. Space allocations (and especially reallocations) that are perceived to be inequitable by faculty can create significant problems (see Chap. 20), so you should use well-understood and standardized policies with metrics and engage your leadership team when making these allocation decisions. Most institutions have metrics and policies for clinical, education, and research space allocation; if yours doesn't or if you are not required to use them, check with peer departments for their models as a reference and work with your leadership team to create ones that are appropriate for your department.

"How Do I Take Space Away from a Faculty Member?"

The criteria for reassignment should be similar for research, clinical, or office space, i.e., inadequate productivity relative to standards that are set by the department and understood by the faculty. Always engage your institutional HR office and departmental leadership team for advice before initiating a process to remove space from a faculty member. Objective documentation and dispassionate evaluation of insufficient productivity is critical in these situations, and you should be prepared for the conflict that may arise (see Chap. 20).

"How Best to Relocate Faculty and Staff into New Space?"

Relocation of faculty and staff often is necessary when the department acquires or loses existing space, programmatic priorities change, there is an opportunity for expansion or consolidation of activities, or there is better proximity to other resources (e.g., equipment, collaborators) that can enhance productivity.

Many questions about new space usually arise when trying to relocate faculty and staff, especially about the timeframe for moving and anticipated extent of downtime. In addition, it is useful to provide information about the new space regarding its relative size, age, configuration, access to equipment and staff support, adjacency to collaborating colleagues, and location on-site or off-site. Unfortunately, in many cases there is resistance to relocation even when the answers to these questions justify the reason for relocation. In such cases, it may be appropriate to consider providing incentives for relocation, including the amount of space assigned, and the resource support provided (e.g., equipment, staff).

Whenever reassigning space, it is important to be sensitive to the concerns of those affected and use productive negotiation (see Chap. 10) to ensure there is a net benefit to all concerned.

Funding

"What Should I Know About Departmental and Institutional Funds Flow?"

As discussed in more detail in the next chapter (Chap. 14), you should meet frequently with the key individuals involved in funds flow and budgeting decisions that impact your department. This includes your own departmental business/financial officer to understand finances from your department's perspective, and your medical school chief financial officer to understand it from the school perspective. It also is important to understand the allocation of support from external sources as applicable, such as your parent university, hospitals, faculty practices, and your state or other governmental entities. Likewise, it is important to know who ultimately approves your overall budget and what you may receive from these other sources.

In brief, funds flow usually is both institution- and department-specific [2–4] and you should understand the following:

- *Ongoing departmental financial commitments*: payment options; flexibility and alternatives such as loans.
- *Departmental reserves*: how they can be accessed and used.
- *Research funding*: distribution of indirect cost recovery for grants; criteria for institutional support.

- *Education income*: institutional support for degree and residency programs; continuing medical education (CME) revenue, tuition; GME funding and distribution.
- *Clinical income*: Medicare part A; relative value unit (RVU) clinical income; criteria for institutional support.
- *Patent/royalty payments*: distribution among the institution, department, and investigators.
- *Philanthropic donations*: institutional overhead; restrictions in accessing donors.
- *Special program funding*: clinical, research, outreach programs, and others.

In evaluating these aspects of funds flow, you should carefully examine sources of income to your department for missed opportunities and determine what expenses are appropriate and how they should be funded, e.g., from operating budget, reserves, and start-up packages. Likewise, you should identify any hidden deficits and obligations, and review long-term financial commitments to determine their need for continuation.

It obviously is important to keep your budget balanced and try to maintain a modest reserve account to handle unanticipated needs. However, you should be careful in accumulating too large a reserve balance because it risks a reduction in institutional support or increased contributions to the institution [5]. It also may result in institutional leadership not helping to fund new programs because your department is perceived to have sufficient funds to do so by itself.

References

1. Taatjes DJ, Chule PN, Bouffard NA, Lee K, DeLance NM, Evans MF. The shared core resource as a partner in innovative scientific research: illustration from an academic microscopy imaging center. J Biomol Tech. 2022;33:1–24. https://doi.org/10.7171/3fc1f5fe.2507f36c.
2. Bailey DN, Crawford JM, Jensen PE, Leonard DGB, McCarthy S, Sanfilippo F. Generating discretionary income in an academic department of pathology. Acad Pathol. 2021;8:23742895211044811. https://doi.org/10.1177/23742895211044811.
3. Itri JN, Mithqal A, Krishnaraj A. Funds flow in the era of value-based health care. J Am Coll Radiol. 2017;14:818–24. https://doi.org/10.1016/j.jacr.2017.01.008.
4. Miller JC, Andersson GE, Cohen M, Cohen SM, Gilbon S, Hindery MA, et al. Follow the money: the implication of medical school's funds flow models. Acad Med. 2012;87:1746–51. https://doi.org/10.1097/ACM.0b013e3182713b77.
5. Winstead DK. Advice for chairs of academic departments of psychiatry: the "ten commandments". Acad Psychiatr. 2006;30:298–300. https://doi.org/10.1176/appi.ap.30.4.298.

Chapter 14
Budgets and Finance

Assessing Departmental Finances

"What Should I Know About My Departmental Finances?"

Three of the most important measures of financial performance that you should understand are:

- Departmental revenue, expenses, and margins (i.e., income statement).
- Assets and liabilities (i.e., balance sheet).
- Cash flow.

Although these are standard items that companies track closely, they often are difficult to assess accurately for medical school departments because of the complex and different cost accounting methods that may be used among programs, departments, and parent and affiliated institutions.

If your parent institutions do not track these measures for your department, it is worth trying to generate your own income statement and balance sheet to monitor finances and plan budgets. For large departments with substantial clinical, research teaching, and public service activities, it is also helpful to track these for your major divisions and sections, with a "roll-up" for your department as a whole.

"What Should I Know About My Institutional Finances?"

As an institutional leader, you should be aware of the bottom line of these three financial measures for your parent institution(s). This will minimize surprises and provide an indication of potential changes in their support. If your institution is running a deficit with low reserves or has cash flow problems, your department could

F. Sanfilippo et al., *Lead, Inspire, Thrive*,
https://doi.org/10.1007/978-3-031-41177-9_14

be affected within a budget cycle. Demonstrating an interest in the financial health of your institution(s) to their leaders is a positive sign of your engagement (see Chap. 28).

"What Should My Department Know About Departmental Finances?"

As discussed above (see Chap. 5, section "Transparency and Establishing Trust"), it is important for members of your department to have trust and confidence in you and the direction of the department. A key to this is for them to know the financial status of the department and institution and how resources are allocated (see Chap. 13). Faculty and departmental meetings and retreats provide good opportunities for you to keep your department informed about finances and resource policies, and answer questions that may come up about either (see Chap. 11, section "Meetings and Events"). Likewise, this information can be conveyed to the department as part of your strategic planning and budget processes and updates, both of which should be transparent and engage departmental members. Limiting the amount of information that you convey about departmental finances can cause unnecessary concern and foster distrust.

"What Institutional Policies Can Affect My Departmental Finances?"

You should be aware of institutional policies that can significantly affect your departmental finances, which may include rules governing:

- *Budgets*: requirements for a specific budgeting process (e.g., zero-based, incremental, see below); submission of a balanced budget; limits on projected margins or deficits; inclusion of a contingency plan.
- *Deficits*: timeframe requirements for resolution; available options, loans.
- *Expenses*: limits or requirements for certain expenditures (e.g., space and equipment leases, contract employees, travel).
- *Income*: institutional "taxes" on revenue from clinical practice, education programs (e.g., CME, GME), philanthropy, and service centers; cost recovery policy for grants; revenue distribution from technology transfer.
- *Margins*: institutional taxes on net margins; limits on how they may be used.
- *Reserves*: restrictions on how they may be invested, spent, or accessed; limits on amount.
- *Support*: processes for institutional funding of departmental activities and related expenses.

Sources and Uses

"How Should I Prioritize Spending?"

Your department may be involved in a wide range of activities that generate expenses (and concomitant income), including clinical and service center programs (revenue), education and training programs (tuition, GME), research and development (grants and contracts), philanthropy (gifts), and technology transfer (payments, equity). Each of these has different rates and timing of return on their expenses, as well as various overhead costs and institutional charges. For example, it is frequently overlooked that research grants actually create significant expenses which are only partially covered by indirect dollars. Programmatically, some of these projects are core mission activities and others are discretionary. Requests for funding support from institutional sources (hospital, medical school, university) are discussed in detail in Chap. 10.

As discussed earlier (Chaps. 2 and 12), spending priorities should be based on the institutional and departmental expectations and strategic initiatives that drive your budget process. Three common issues that are often difficult to resolve are:

- How to distribute support among programmatic priorities?
- How much support should be provided for overhead to facilitate program success?
- How much funding should go to low-priority activities which generate net margins that can be used to support high-priority activities?

Distributing support across strategic program priorities is often difficult because there rarely are enough resources to meet the needs and opportunities for all of them in a single budget cycle. A useful approach is creating a timeline to be sure each of the priorities receives support during the timeframe of your strategic plan. Letting program leaders know that the resources they need will vary across the timing of the strategic plan can help reduce the tension among priority program leaders. It also can enhance collaboration among program priorities by preferentially providing resources to activities that span multiple program priorities.

Evaluating your overhead (indirect) expenses relative to program activity (direct) expenses is a useful indicator of efficiency. Comparisons with aspirational peer departments can be helpful, but since costs for space and support staff can vary significantly by region, it may be more useful to compare your overhead expenses with high-performing units of similar size and activity at your own institution.

Funding low-priority programs that generate greater net margins to support high-priority programs can create significant problems with faculty and other stakeholders involved in both types of programs, and sends conflicting messages to your department. Cross-subsidies are common in most institutions, with the clinical enterprise often subsidizing the academic missions of education and research. Nonetheless, such subsidies are always controversial, whether within or between departments. For that reason, so-called "mission-based" budgeting was developed for medical schools years ago whereby costs and activities are aligned by mission [1], but few institutions still use this model. It is often better to support additional revenue-generating activities, such as philanthropic fundraising, within departmental priority program areas. High-priority programs always should be challenged to identify activities that could generate additional support.

"How Can I Be Flexible with Expenses?"

Depending on the state of your current and projected income, reserves, and cash flow, there are various ways to adjust expenses to help your financial standing. For administrative activities, using contracted staff and consultants rather than full-time employees can provide flexibility and potential cost-savings. Employees also can be hired as part-time with either limited to no benefits, or as flex-time, depending upon the workload. Likewise, the use of part-time contract faculty or fellows rather than full-time faculty can provide financial benefits while maintaining productivity. However, the financial benefits may be offset by diminished engagement, productivity, and control, as well as unintended and undesirable consequences to departmental culture, quality of training experiences, collaboration, and collegiality (see Chaps. 6 and 8).

At most AHCs/AMCs, the compensation level can vary significantly between tenure track faculty and those on non-tenure clinical, research, or teaching tracks. Expanding the use of clinical, research, and teaching fellows may mitigate the need for additional faculty. In many cases the expense for "buying-out" (e.g., early retirement) a full-time, tenured, but poorly productive faculty member may be beneficial to the overall financial health and productivity of the department, especially considering net-present values and opportunity costs. Again, these approaches may have unanticipated or undesired consequences, especially in terms of departmental culture.

Depending on your institutional policies, financial options also may be available when considering space and equipment expenses. Renting space (versus purchasing), and leasing equipment (versus buying), may provide substantial financial benefits and desirable effects on your cash flow, income statement, and balance sheet. For example, renting space or leasing equipment may be preferable when you have good income and cash flow, but low reserves and a weak balance sheet.

Developing a Budget

"What Is the Best Budget Process for My Department?"

Your budget and budget process should be closely tied to your strategic plan and are essential mechanisms for increasing efficiency and productivity. In many ways the budget is a roadmap to guide you toward achieving your department's goals [2]. While there are several different budget processes, most boil down to being either incremental (updating and building on an existing budget) or zero-based (starting from scratch).

Incremental budgeting is the easiest and most common approach to budgeting and appropriate when there are no significant projected changes in expenses, income, and priorities [3]. However, the major problems with this approach are perpetuating errors and missing opportunities. Budgets that have been in place for a long period with small incremental annual changes tend to receive a cursory review and become thought of as entitlements, resulting in less motivation to reduce expenses and increase revenue.

In contrast, zero-based budgeting requires justification in each budget cycle of all the projected income and expenses that are related to each activity. It is most appropriate when there are significant anticipated changes in priorities and activities (e.g., resulting from a new strategic plan) or environmental changes that would significantly affect income or expenses. Zero-based budgeting requires much greater time and effort, but usually provides a greater degree of transparency and engagement of faculty and staff [4].

In many cases, the best approach for budgeting is a combination of incremental budgeting for high-performing programs anticipating little change and zero-based budgeting for programs that have not performed well, are undergoing substantial changes (e.g., new leadership), or are newly developed.

"What Assumptions Should I Make When Budgeting?"

Regardless of the type of budget process utilized, your assumptions about income and expenses are dependent on numerous institutional and environmental factors, which ultimately will determine your budget and therefore your program allocations. There usually is a wide variation in the extent and accuracy of the stringency analyses needed for different assumptions, which can substantially affect the time and effort of budgeting as well as the extent of contingency planning.

The appropriate level of detail for assessing the income and expense assumptions of different budget components is influenced by several factors including financial magnitude, economic trends, program importance, anticipated changes in policy and payments, and fiscal health. For budget components requiring significant accuracy of assumptions, outside expert advisors or consultants may be needed (see Chap. 34).

Margins and Deficits

"How Should I Use Unexpected Financial Margins?"

There often are institutional policies on how net margins can be used, and, in any case, this is always a good problem. When new funds are available for discretionary use, your first consideration should be to assess your department's overall financial health. For example, if you have a weak balance sheet, it may be advisable to increase your reserve funds. Alternatively, if you are in strong financial shape, you may consider increasing the funding of high-priority programs, supporting infrastructure to facilitate productivity, or seeding a new program of great potential. In all cases, you should engage and be transparent with your departmental and institutional leadership and follow the priorities of your strategic plan [5].

"How Should I Deal with an Unexpected Financial Deficit?"

Not meeting your budget is a difficult problem for you, your department, and the institution and usually reflects inaccurate assumptions of income or expenses. In most cases, your institutions will have policies on how unbudgeted deficits are to be handled, since they will be directly affected by the shortfall. Therefore, it is wise to alert institutional leadership as soon as deficits are anticipated, so appropriate contingency planning can be considered. In some rare cases intra- or extra-institutional loans may be required, depending upon the magnitude of the deficit. In addition, you should be sure departmental faculty and staff, as well as key stakeholders, are appropriately made aware of the problem and the potential plans for dealing with it.

As with unanticipated margins, a good first step in dealing with unexpected deficits is evaluating the department's financial health to consider options such as reducing reserves or program activities or, if allowed, incurring a penalty to carry the deficit. A critically important step is to evaluate how the deficit occurred and what assumptions were inaccurate, so they can be more carefully evaluated in the next budget process and explained to all key stakeholders (faculty, staff, donors, community leaders), including institutional leadership when they question the deficit.

Remember, whether a margin or deficit, institutional leaders consider it their money, so engage them early and minimize surprises!

References

1. Sainte M, Kanter SL, Muller D. Mission-based budgeting for education: ready for prime time? Mt Sinai J Med. 2009;76:381–6. https://doi.org/10.1002/msj.20122.
2. Ross TK. Budgeting for results. Health Care Manag. 2020;39:24–34. https://doi.org/10.1097/HCM.0000000000000285.
3. Schick AG, Hills FS. Size, stability and incremental budgeting outcomes in public universities. J Manage. 1982;8:49–64. https://doi.org/10.1177/014920638200800204.
4. Coyte R, Messner M, Zhou S. The revival of zero-based budgeting: drivers and consequences of firm-level adoptions. Account Finance. 2021;62:3147–88. https://doi.org/10.1111/acfi.12884.
5. Bailey DN, Crawford JM, Jensen PE, Leonard DGB, McCarthy S, Sanfilippo F. Generating discretionary income in an academic department of pathology. Acad Pathol. 2021;8:23742895211044811. https://doi.org/10.1177/23742895211044811.

Chapter 15
Balancing the Missions

The Balancing Act

"How Do I Successfully Balance the Research, Clinical, Education, and Public Service Missions of the Department?"

Faculty generally excel in one or two mission areas and few can excel at four (education, clinical, research, and public service), the so-called quadripartite mission. Thus, your challenge is to have faculty and staff distributed appropriately in programmatic areas and able to collaborate effectively to meet expectations across all your department's missions and priorities. In at least one report, questions about balancing the missions were among the most frequently posed by department chairs [1]; balancing your department's mission will be critical to your success [2].

Given the heterogeneity of medical school faculty, most institutions have developed a wide range of tenure and non-tenured faculty tracks, which include various combinations of clinical, research, and educator pathways. It is incumbent for you to understand these tracks at your institution and ensure that faculty are placed into the one most appropriate for them to flourish with the necessary mentorship (see Chap. 18). Regardless of the academic track assigned, you should make sure that all faculty are engaged in teaching and some type of service to the department and institution (e.g., administrative role, committee work, community outreach).

It is also important that each of your department's mission activities has established metrics for evaluation such as teaching hours and student evaluations, publications and citations, research grants, work RVUs, patient satisfaction surveys, honors and awards, and committee participation. This requires that faculty maintain up-to-date documentation of their activities in each area.

An important part of your responsibilities as leader is to ensure that overall departmental goals, as well as individual faculty goals, are set for each mission area.

F. Sanfilippo et al., *Lead, Inspire, Thrive*, https://doi.org/10.1007/978-3-031-41177-9_15

An important way to achieve balance across missions is to have strong collaboration among faculty, especially between research and clinical faculty (see Chap. 8).

Your Involvement in Each Mission

"To What Extent Should I as Leader Be Directly Engaged in Clinical Service, Research, and Teaching, Given My Administrative Duties and Responsibilities?"

As leader of your department and to establish and maintain credibility with your faculty, you should be engaged to some extent in each mission area and strive to maintain productivity in as many as possible. You also should try to synergize your activities across mission areas, especially in collaboration with other departments and centers across your AHC/AMC and university, as a role model to your faculty of how they can collaborate and be aligned (see below).

Being active across mission areas also ensures that you will have future opportunities upon transitioning from your leadership role, especially if you choose to remain as a faculty member in the department you now lead (see Chap. 37). Maintaining such activity is easier if you were recruited internally and already have educational, clinical, research, and service activities established. It is much harder to re-establish all your activities when moving to another institution in a leadership role, which is why many externally recruited department chairs cut back on activity in one or more mission areas.

Alignment of Missions

"How Can I Ensure That the Missions of My Department Are Properly Aligned?"

Alignment of missions is important for faculty and for the department overall. However, it is difficult for a faculty member to have clinical expertise in one area and be required to teach in a very different area. Misalignment can lead to poor faculty productivity and morale. In fact, a major reason that clinical faculty leave academic practice has been attributed to difficulty in balancing competing demands and institutional expectations [3].

Moreover, at most AHCs/AMCs, clinical revenues subsidize education and research, especially because of the common funding shortfalls for the latter two [4]. Dependence upon such subsidies places those two mission areas at risk due to increasing institutional restrictions on use of clinical revenue for purposes other than supporting clinical faculty and activities. Such cross-subsidies also can create friction with the clinical faculty who generate the clinical revenue. This can result in more pressure upon faculty to generate funds for their research and education activities, as well as for the department and institution to provide (and fund) protected time for the academic activities of clinical faculty.

Despite these issues, there are several potential ways to align the missions of your department. Your strategic plan should have goals and priorities for each mission with ways to leverage programs across missions and disciplines [5] (see Chap. 12). Similarly, your budget and budget process should leverage resource allocations among programs to support your strategic plan and tactics to achieve expectations across missions. At the faculty level, you should help ensure that the clinical activity of faculty informs their teaching as well as scholarly activities, which can promote their productivity across missions. Likewise, facilitating collaboration among your faculty across mission areas within your department and with institutional programs and centers can help align and expand your research and clinical missions (see Chaps. 8, section "Research and Clinical Faculty Relationships" and 13, section "People"). And as mentioned above, your own engagement and activity across missions provides a strong message to your faculty and staff about the importance of aligning and leveraging departmental missions.

References

1. Bailey DN, Cohen S, Gotlieb A, Lipscomb MF, Sanfilippo F. What advice current pathology chairs seek from former chairs. Acad Pathol. 2018;5:2374289518807397. https://doi.org/10.1177/2374289518807397.
2. Ness RB, Samet JM. How to be a department chair of epidemiology: a survival guide. Am J Epidemiol. 2010;172:747–51. https://doi.org/10.1093/aje/kwq268.
3. Girod SC, Fassioto M, Menorca R, Etzkowitz H, Wren SM. Reasons or faculty departures from an academic medical center: a survey and comparison across faculty lines. BMC Med Educ. 2017;17:8. https://doi.org/10.1186/s12909-016-0830-y.
4. Rawson JV, Baron RL. Balancing the three missions and the impact on academic radiology. Acad Radiol. 2013;20:1190–4. https://doi.org/10.1016/j.acra.2013.04.003.
5. Gonzalo JD, Dekhtyar M, Caverzagie KJ, Grant BK, Herrine SK, Nussbaum AM, et al. The triple helix of clinical, research, and education missions in academic health centers: a qualitative study of diverse stakeholder perspectives. Learn Health Syst. 2021;5:e10250. https://doi.org/10.1002/lrh2.10250.

Chapter 16
Crisis Management

General

"How Should I Deal with a Significant and Unexpected Crisis in My Department?"

When dealing with a crisis, you should use your departmental leadership to create a "crisis management team" focused on consequences, immediate responses, and sustainable solutions. Although there are many types of crises, they all are time-sensitive, pose significant risks, and require consequential decisions [1, 2].

Communication should be at the very heart of crisis management. It will facilitate coordination as well as provide reassurance to faculty, staff, and students and trainees. Your behavior and emotional response to any crisis is an important role model and sets the tone for others. Communicate issues and planned resolution with institutional leaders; be transparent and try to avoid surprises [3]! Get advice and help as needed from institutional leaders, peers, and outside experts (see Chap. 34).

The onset of a crisis can be sudden with little or no time for planning, in contrast to crises that are anticipated or develop gradually, which provide more time to plan for contingencies. Likewise, it is important to anticipate if the crisis will be short-lived or ongoing to plan accordingly. Occasionally, a crisis may be compounded (e.g., a pandemic resulting in financial, personal, and staffing crises), requiring you to set priorities on how to handle the multiple crises as well as basic operations.

Financial

"What Should I Do If My Department Has a Significant and Unexpected Budget Problem?"

The first step in dealing with a serious budget problem is to identify the cause and determine the impact (see Chap. 13, section "Funding" and Chap. 14, section "Margins and Deficits"). For problems that are internal to your department, establish whether they are due to revenue shortfalls (e.g., decreased clinical activity, grant funding, reimbursement, philanthropy), increased expenses (e.g., staffing, infrastructure, supplies-equipment), or both. For problems that are institutional, again determine whether they are due to revenue shortfalls (e.g., decreased allocations from the school or health system), increased expenses (e.g., increased "dean's tax"), or a combination of both.

Having categorized the cause of a shortfall, you then should determine whether it will be ongoing or a one-time event. Resolution of an acute problem can often be made with quick fixes, while chronic problems usually require more major structural changes. Evaluate consequences and potential solutions with your departmental leadership team, and discuss the approaches you plan to use with institutional leadership for input before implementation. Consider negotiating with institutional leadership to address the problem by proposing more institutional support to help replace departmental shortfalls and partial deferment or reduction of institutional cuts if the shortfall has an institutional etiology (see Chap. 10).

Environmental

"How Should I Prioritize Activities During an Environmental Crisis?"

Since an environmental crisis will normally impact the entire institution and beyond, institutional and community issues must take priority over departmental ones. Types of environmental crises include natural disasters (e.g., hurricanes, tornadoes, floods, fires, heat/cold waves), pandemics, accidents, and incidents.

Natural disasters are the most common type of environmental crisis and are usually short-lived, although the aftermath can take a while to resolve. Furthermore, they often are local occurrences, with outside help available (e.g., Federal Emergency Management Authority, American Red Cross). Accidents and incidents (e.g., transportation-related such as airplane crashes, facility-related such as building collapse or fire, targeted physical or cyberattacks) are one-time events for which contingency plans are often in place. Civil disturbances may be more variable in their scope and duration, while pandemics are often regional, national, and even international in nature with an unpredictable course that may be prolonged.

Your parent institution(s) will have general (and in some cases specific) crisis management procedures available, in addition to the federal, state, and municipal plans, that will provide direction for your response. Make sure your departmental response is fully aligned with institutional and governmental policies and processes. Immediately notify your institution's crisis management team if their direction to you or your department is ambiguous or potentially counter-productive.

The biggest problem with environmental crises usually is maintaining staffing levels to meet demands. It is essential to identify the most critical services needed and how to reallocate staff. Consider appropriate rationing of services and assess its impact with your leadership team, and engage institutional leadership before implementation.

Personal

"How Should I Prioritize My Activities During a Personal Crisis?"

When faced with a personal crisis, you should assess the severity and potential length of disruption and its impact on the amount and quality of time you can devote to your department. Acute personal health issues may be relatively short-lived, while chronic and life-threatening illnesses will have more serious and sustained impact on your ability to lead the department. Although illness of a family member or financial problems can be very distracting, you may be able to adjust the time commitment needed to deal with these types of personal crises through long-term planning.

As appropriate, discuss personal crises and their potential impact with your leadership team, and solicit advice and assistance from all available sources (see Chap. 34). Options can include delegating more authority to departmental leaders and considering a leave of absence or sick leave. If your ability to carry out your job is compromised, you should discuss options with your institutional leaders before acting.

Opportunities to Learn from Crises

"What Lessons Can Be Learned from Crises?"

While no leader wishes for crises to occur, when they do, they almost always provide useful lessons that test and enhance leadership skills. These include appreciating the resilience and flexibility of your team; understanding the importance of communication; valuing the significance of remaining calm; taking time to frame issues, plan, and implement solutions; and making transformational changes [4].

You should always look for new opportunities that can emerge from a crisis. In many cases a crisis allows significant transformational changes to be made that otherwise could not be accomplished as rapidly or at all (see Chap. 12, section "Managing Change"). Several examples of this have resulted from the recent COVID pandemic in each mission area, such as the increased use of virtual classes, greater use of telehealth consultations, and more rapid translation of research to clinical application. Operational changes also resulted from the pandemic, especially regarding staffing shortages, which led to more flexibility for working from home, job cross-coverage, and virtual meetings [5]. As often credited to Winston Churchill, "Never let a good crisis go to waste!"

References

1. Kaiser RB. Leading in an unprecedented global crisis: the heightened importance of versatility. Consult Psychol J. 2020;72:135–54. https://doi.org/10.1037/cpb0000186.
2. Oroszi T. A preliminary analysis of high-stakes decision-making for crisis leadership. J Bus Contin Emer Plan. 2018;11:335–59. PMID 30670135.
3. Eldridge CC, Hampton D, Marfell J. Communication during crisis. Nurs Manag. 2020;51:50–3. https://doi.org/10.1097/01.NUMA.0000688976.29383.dc.
4. Glotzbecker MP. Crisis leadership: lessons learned from the COVID pandemic. J Pediatr Orthop. 2022;42(Suppl 1):S56–9. https://doi.org/10.1097/BPO.0000000000002068.
5. Kaul V. Leadership during crisis: lessons and applications from the COVID-19 pandemic. Gastroenterology. 2020;159:809–12. https://doi.org/10.1053/j.gastro.2020.04.076.

Part IV
Faculty Issues

An essential asset that ultimately will determine success for you and your department is the productivity and achievements of your faculty. Recruitment and retention of faculty members who enhance the performance and culture of your department are critical factors, as is providing them with an environment and resources that facilitate their accomplishments. Implementing programs to enhance the career development and wellness of faculty should be a high priority, as well as providing competitive compensation and constructive performance reviews. Dealing appropriately with faculty who are nonproductive or disruptive is essential for maintaining your department's stability and well-being and is one of the greatest challenges for every department chair.

Chapter 17
Faculty Recruitment and Retention

Recruiting New Faculty

"When and How Should I Start a Search for a New Faculty Member?"

Generally, there are two types of recruitments: (1) demand-driven (i.e., to fill a specific departmental need or to expand a programmatic area) and (2) opportunity-driven (i.e., to take advantage of an opportunity that would add value to the department). The former should take priority, especially if the need is to fill an existing position that has become vacant, while the second is optional and normally requires the use of discretionary resources.

Questions you should be ready to answer when recruiting an individual to fill an existing faculty position include:

- How flexible is the existing position? Will it be a good fit for the new recruit?
- Why is the existing position vacant? Is it because of problems (e.g., too much work, not enough support, bad environment, problem co-workers or supervisor)?
- How are the salary and related expenses of the existing position budgeted? Are the sources stable and ongoing?

Questions you should be ready to answer when recruiting to a newly created position include:

- Why was the position created?
- How well defined and flexible are the roles, authority, and responsibilities of the position?
- Is the position due to an expansion of an existing program or the start of a new one?

© The Author(s), under exclusive license to Springer Nature
Switzerland AG 2023

F. Sanfilippo et al., *Lead, Inspire, Thrive*,
https://doi.org/10.1007/978-3-031-41177-9_17

In any type of faculty recruitment, the professional interests and activities of the candidate should fit well with the faculty and programs of the department and institution. Likewise, the candidate should fit well with the culture of the department and institution and be a good potential team player. It also is worth engaging institutional leadership in important faculty recruitments, especially those in other departments and centers/institutes that involve the candidate's interests and discipline. This helps send a positive message to the candidates, keeps leadership informed of program development, and increases the potential of additional support for the recruitment (see Chap. 13, section "People").

You always should try to discover why an individual wants to leave their current position; some reasons make good sense while others should be a red flag. It is not unusual for high-performing faculty to look for new positions when their resources become insufficient or there is a change in leadership that does not appreciate their value. In many cases a candidate may recognize a greater potential opportunity in your department for advancement, flexibility, or productivity. Another attraction may be the prestige of your institution and department, especially in their area of interest, and the higher quality of your students, residents, and fellows: the best trainees attract the best faculty and vice versa [1]. However, in some cases individuals look at new positions to create a bidding war for a large retention package at their home institution or to use a position simply to get more resources as a stepping-stone before they look for a subsequent position with even more resources, without a true commitment to the department that is recruiting them.

When faced with multiple attractive candidates, you should consider the relative benefits and disadvantages of more junior versus senior candidates. Junior candidates often require fewer resources and less salary and are more flexible. Senior candidates potentially have more experience, can bring or quickly build a group or program, and often have more connections with your departmental faculty. In most cases, senior candidates will usually require more resources, including space, staff support, and compensation.

Similarly, there are advantages and disadvantages in recruiting internal (e.g., those finishing training) versus external candidates. Internal candidates, and those with previous experience at your institution, know the culture and members of your institution, know the local and regional environment, are more likely to be a good fit with a quicker transition into the position, and already may have significant ongoing clinical and research collaborations at your institution. In contrast, external candidates potentially can bring new views, ideas, activities, and collaborators.

When recruiting new faculty, you should consider whether or not the position might best be jointly recruited with another department, center, or institute in your AHC/AMC or even on the general university campus. Not only may this assist your department financially, but also it may build important interdisciplinary bridges for your department and may help to recruit uniquely qualified candidates (see Chap. 13, section "People").

"Should I Use a Search Firm?"

There are several factors to consider when deciding whether or not to use a search firm for recruitment of a faculty member. Although there is a significant financial cost for using a search firm, this should be weighed against the anticipated savings in the time and effort for you and your department, as well as the potential benefits of their assistance.

One of the major benefits that search firms can provide is by using their experience and network of past and current candidates to identify a larger pool of potential candidates than you might be able to find. Search firms often play a particularly important role in identifying a more diverse pool of candidates (see Chap. 7). These consultants can save time and expense and may be especially useful when trying to recruit senior and highly specialized faculty, or a group of faculty together as a clinical or research team. In addition, search firms often know of potential candidates who wish to remain highly confidential and would not respond to open solicitations.

Another potential benefit of search firms is their experience and expertise in screening, vetting, and communicating candidly with potential candidates as well as those asked to provide references. As your consultants, they also can be very helpful as intermediaries in negotiating agreement terms with candidates, which can help avoid misunderstandings and even contentious disagreements between you and a future faculty or staff member in your department.

"What Best Practices Are Recommended for Appointing Search Committees?"

You should carefully consider whom to appoint to your search committee for new faculty hires. Choose committee members who have a track record of working for the department's success and who won't bring their personal agendas to their decision-making. A diversity of perspectives and expertise are highly desirable, and the search committee should reflect the breadth of the department. Particular attention should be paid to including women and those from underrepresented groups (while avoiding gender or minority "taxes" of service overload). All search committee members should have training in unconscious and other forms of bias [2]. Committees should be instructed that slates of recommended candidates that fail to include women and those from historically excluded groups in medicine will not be accepted (see Chap. 7) [3, 4].

"What Start-Up Resources Should I Consider for New Faculty?"

One of the challenges you face in recruitment is finding the best person that can be attracted to the position with the resources available. Your department should have a standardized recruitment process that includes creating the recruitment plan, developing and posting notices about the position, conducting interviews, evaluating candidates, selecting candidates, and making the offer.

The size of start-up resources ("packages") for research and clinical faculty varies by institution and department and typically is determined by the roles, responsibilities, seniority, and the stature of the individual being recruited. For research faculty, most institutions use grant dollars/square foot as a method to determine appropriate space, equipment, and staff support. For clinical faculty, resources typically involve defined access to appropriate inpatient, outpatient, and office facilities, along with equipment and staff support. In some cases, recruitment packages are largely determined prior to the search, while in others the package is tailored to the specific needs and expectations of the candidate and the department. In all cases, compensation should be based on benchmarks and productivity measures as established in your department's compensation plan (see Chap. 19).

You should know if your institution has policies or criteria about what can and cannot be offered to recruits, especially regarding perks such as signing bonuses, parking, reimbursed memberships, etc., which can become the tipping point for a successful recruitment. You also should explain to recruits any department or institution policies on how start-up funds may be expended, and particularly if they are allowed to be banked for future use if not expended in the timeframe expected. In setting annual performance criteria for recruited faculty, be sure to include their use of the start-up resources that were provided in the context of their progress and accomplishments. Occasionally faculty will underspend their package to hang on to resources at the expense of their productivity.

One approach in recruiting talent is to decide beforehand what attributes you are seeking (e.g., senior versus junior faculty member, the specific talents desired) and the resources (funding, space, equipment, staff support) you are willing and able to offer. Screening candidates becomes easier with those attributes and resources in mind. However, if your criteria become too narrow, you may be eliminating potential candidates who might fit your position very well and be worth the added resource expenditure.

"What Are Effective Ways to Interact with Candidates?"

An important part of successful recruitment is for you to develop a personal rapport with faculty being recruited to your department. Even if a search is being led by another member of your department and your future interactions will be modest, most recruits realize that their success ultimately is dependent on your support for resources and promotion and will value your personal involvement in their recruitment. You should take advantage of opportunities to spend private time with recruits that includes discussion about their family, hobbies, and personal interests. Occasional phone calls and virtual meetings also will make a substantial impression on recruits.

Another useful recruitment tactic, especially for public searches, is to visit the finalist candidate(s) you are trying to recruit at their institution, at which time you can discuss the components of an offer on their turf. Such an offer to visit them will flatter recruits and hopefully put them at ease, while you will be able to see the environments in which they work. If a finalist candidate is not interested in your visiting them, be sure to find out why. For searches that are not public, it simply may be a matter of wanting to maintain local confidentiality until an agreement is reached, or not wanting to upset their students and colleagues. Or it may be a red flag that they are not really interested in the position or not well regarded at their institution. If they are interested, they can make their subsequent interview visit an implicit acceptance of the offer.

"What Should I Consider When Onboarding New Faculty Recruits?"

A key to the success of a newly recruited faculty member is their transition into your department. Even for those who have been at your institution previously as students or faculty, coming into your department provides a new set of expectations, resources, opportunities, and interactions with faculty, students, and staff.

At most institutions, your HR department will provide an orientation program to familiarize new faculty with institutional processes, compliance requirements, available human resources and programs, and other logistical issues. However, it is up to you and your department to provide an effective means of having new faculty members feel comfortable with expectations in their new role, understand the culture and behavioral norms of their new environment, and become an engaged member of their new department.

An excellent way to facilitate the transition of new faculty is by developing a formal or informal onboarding program that includes providing information about the department and its policies and practices, scheduling meetings with key members of the faculty and staff, answering questions, and assigning faculty advisors/mentors to help with professional development and career guidance (see Chap. 18, section "Implementing Career Development Programs").

Retaining Current Talent

"What Are Effective Strategies for Retaining Faculty Who Consider Leaving Your Department?"

There are many factors involved in deciding whether or not to try to retain a faculty member who is contemplating leaving your department. Retention strategies are dependent upon the ability of your department and institution(s) to make a counter-offer, what is driving the faculty member to leave (e.g., greater compensation, more space, support staff, and equipment, a higher leadership position), and the potential costs of losing the individual. In some cases, the cost of having to replace productive faculty members in lost effort and recruitment expenses will far outweigh the resources needed to successfully retain them.

If you find that faculty who are valuable to the department are considering other opportunities, you should check on the programs and processes you have in place to help them be successful and satisfied in their career development and personal wellness (see Chap. 18). Often, the need to retain good faculty identifies the need to improve these programs, which can reduce the likelihood of additional retention efforts. Retention of talented faculty may also be facilitated by engaging other departments and centers in your medical school, AHC/AMC, and university, particularly if your faculty member provides special value to the other units.

If it appears that an alternative position being considered by a faculty member would provide better career development opportunities, you should be supportive of their decision to leave. This will demonstrate to your faculty that you are most interested in their success. However, be aware of game-playing by faculty members who may be trying to obtain additional resources from the department by threatening to leave. If the outside recruitment is serious and it makes the most sense to try to retain the individual, your attempts at retention should begin sooner rather than later to have the best chance of being successful. In any case, you should never get into bidding wars over the retention (or recruitment) of faculty.

Closing the Deal

"What Are Some of the Issues I Should Consider to Be Successful in Faculty Recruitment and Retention?"

Some of the recruitment/retention issues to consider in addition to the start-up package and perks mentioned above include education-related debt, availability of experienced and effective mentors, career guidance, access to resources to help develop grant proposals, teaching and presentation skills, and protected time for research and other academic pursuits [5].

You always should remember that you are recruiting/retaining a family and not just a person. Pay attention to their spouse's or partner's job, children's schools, parents' health, cost and availability of desired housing, etc. These are often make or break issues. Be proactive in addressing these issues and ready to provide contacts for schools and realtors, especially if they are issues in your geographic area. Paying attention to all of the little details will help make the individual feel wanted. Frequent and attentive communication is key, and all concerns and questions of the faculty member you are trying to recruit or retain should be taken seriously and addressed to their full satisfaction [1].

Perhaps the most important aspect in finalizing the recruitment or retention of a faculty member is to avoid contentious negotiation of their compensation or resource package (see Chap. 10). For new faculty, it may be best to have the components of an offer discussed through an intermediary who is trusted by both parties, such as the chair of the search committee or a search consultant. For department faculty you are trying to retain, this can be done by their direct supervisor or leader of their division/unit or a member of your senior leadership team, especially your vice chair for faculty affairs or equivalent.

"Should I Make a Special Deal to Recruit or Retain a Special or Extraordinary Individual?"

There is substantial risk in changing policy or standards to address a special situation, whether for an extraordinary recruitment opportunity, the perfect candidate for an important vacant position, or to retain a very valuable faculty or staff member. These risks include jealousy of other faculty members ("why not me?"), perception by other faculty that policy/standards do not apply equally to everyone (which can lead them to challenge other policies and standards), belief by the recruited/retained faculty member that policy/standards don't apply to them (which usually creates problems at some later point), and a concern by institutional leaders that you are making exceptions for some faculty but not others (which can damage your credibility with them). Any changes to policy or standards that you might consider in such circumstances should be fully vetted beforehand with appropriate members of your department and institutional leaders to understand the potential opportunities and risks involved.

Appointments, Promotions, and Tenure

"What Should I Know About the Faculty Appointments, Promotions, and Tenure (APT) Process at My Institution?"

An important consideration with faculty recruitment and retention is the APT process at your institution, which you should understand fully. Many AHCs/AMCs now have multiple pathways (tracks) to which faculty may be appointed, usually based on the mission area in which the majority of their work and scholarship will be focused (e.g., clinical, research, education). In most cases, only some of the tracks are tenured. You should understand the various tracks used at your school and the expectations for faculty in each of the tracks to ensure that they are in the track which best reflects their role (see Chap. 15). In addition, if your institution allows accelerated promotion or merit advancement you should be aware of these policies and apply them equitably.

An occasional issue with faculty appointments can arise if faculty members are permitted to change faculty tracks at your institution. Such requests may be initiated by the faculty member or be the result of advice you provide, especially when a valuable faculty member is not likely to achieve tenure within the time specified by the university and requests reappointment to a non-tenure clinical, education, or research track. Switching tracks, especially because of inadequate performance in meeting the expectations of the original track, should be discouraged except when there has been a deliberate re-definition of the faculty member's role.

The APT process can vary substantially among medical schools and universities, but in almost all cases begins at the departmental level with a review of the candidate by a standing or ad hoc group of faculty who are at the same or higher academic rank. It is important to know if there is a standard policy set by your institution for departmental reviews and how much flexibility (if any) is available. The process may differ by the track and rank (e.g., instructor, assistant, associate, professor) being considered for the appointment or promotion.

You also should understand the processes subsequent to the departmental review. In most cases the departmental review for APT will be given to you with a recommendation, and you must decide whether to agree or disagree. To move forward, the review and recommendations by you and the department typically are submitted to a medical school APT committee for similar review and, if positive, then submitted to the university APT committee with ultimate approval vested in the Board of Trustees or a similar governing body.

"What Are Some Issues That Can Arise with Faculty Appointments?"

Determining the appropriate rank and track of a new faculty appointment is part of the recruitment process, and in many cases the departmental search committee can be used as a surrogate for the departmental APT committee to bring forward your candidate for appointment to the medical school and university. It is always important to remind candidates that their appointment is not finalized until approved by your institution's governance board.

In many instances, hospitals that are affiliated with (or owned by) a university may have a closed medical staff, requiring a faculty appointment for clinical privileges. Occasionally, this may create a problem with the timing needs of the candidate and hospital, especially since appointments are not final until they have gone through the appropriate APT committees and receive board approval. If this is a problem at your institution, you should work with other chairs and your institutional leadership to develop an appropriate expedient process to deal with such situations. In some institutions such individuals may be placed onto an employment contract (as a staff physician) prior to receiving their formal academic appointments.

"What Are Some Issues That Can Arise with Faculty Promotions and Tenure?"

Disagreement with the recommendation of your departmental APT committee regarding the promotion or tenure of a faculty member is a serious issue and will be difficult for you to handle with the committee and the faculty member involved, as well as the medical school. However, disagreements occasionally occur, especially when the promotion or tenure criteria are ambiguous, or if you came from an institution where they were significantly different, or if you are concerned about subtle or personal bias by anyone on the committee (see Chap. 7). In such cases, you should have a candid discussion with your departmental APT committee over the disagreements to determine their position and work quickly to resolve any issues. Subsequently, you should discuss the situation with the faculty member.

If you decided against a positive recommendation by the committee, you should be well prepared and get advice from your institutional offices of faculty affairs as well as legal counsel before meeting with the candidate. These situations can result in a lawsuit against you and the institution if the faculty member feels they were treated unfairly.

In cases where the departmental APT committee recommended against promotion or tenure, but you wish to proceed, you should follow a similar process of discussion with the APT committee and then the faculty member. If your institution allows you to bring forward candidates not recommended by your APT committee, you should be well prepared to justify your support to the institutional committees.

"What About Clinical Faculty Who Are Hospital Employees?"

In some AHCs/AMCs, especially larger ones, physicians may be needed to provide clinical service with minimal, if any, teaching and essentially no scholarly expectations. These individuals are often hired on employment contracts with the hospital or their associated clinics and are not paid through faculty salary lines, but may receive direct or indirect compensation for their service to the medical school. They will frequently work side by side with your faculty who are paid through faculty salary lines and will often interact with your students and trainees. In addition, they customarily have different salary structures (and perhaps even larger salaries) than your other clinical faculty who must address the multiple missions of the medical school.

Clinical staff physicians who are not salaried faculty and normally employed by the hospital (not the medical school) usually are not allowed to vote on faculty matters. These differences can create tension among the faculty and even their trainees. In many institutions, such contracted physicians may be given "volunteer" or "adjunct" clinical faculty titles in attempt to mitigate misunderstandings and recognize their interaction with students and trainees (see above). As department chair it is important that you be keenly aware of these differences and make every attempt to minimize tension with these hospital- or clinic-based employed staff physicians (with or without volunteer faculty titles), and try to optimize the benefits they can provide.

"What About Emeriti Faculty and Volunteer Faculty?"

Retired faculty (sometimes given the title of "emeritus," depending upon institutional policy) are often eager to continue their participation in the department. In most cases this is done without compensation and can be a useful way for the department to obtain additional faculty support without impacting the budget. At some institutions, retired and emeriti faculty can return part-time (designated "recall" at some AHCs/AMCs) and receive compensation in addition to their retirement pay.

Regardless of whether they are compensated, emeriti faculty frequently fill valuable teaching roles for medical students, graduate students, and house staff. Because they have retired from your department, they know the department's organization, culture, and people and do not need to be brought up to speed. Occasionally, such individuals may also perform clinical activities if they have maintained their clinical privileges in the hospital and clinics. In those instances, they may wish to be compensated on a part-time basis (without benefits because they are retired) if allowed by institutional policy and if those activities generate clinical revenue that is at least sufficient to cover their earnings.

Apart from these retired faculty, individuals at other institutions including industry and affiliated universities and health-care facilities often desire to volunteer their expertise, in return for which they receive volunteer faculty titles (e.g., volunteer/visiting/adjunct professor). These individuals can be particularly helpful in the educational mission, and in some instances, they may also provide clinical service in areas of shortage. In the latter cases, they must meet criteria for and maintain clinical staff privileges at the hospital/clinic and may seek some compensation reflecting revenues generated by their work. Because they do not have faculty salary lines, they may need to be employed via a contract coupled with a volunteer faculty appointment if they wish to provide clinical care.

It is important to recognize such emeriti and volunteer faculty by hosting "thank-you" events and inviting them to department social gatherings. In addition to both groups providing valuable support to your department with little or no monetary cost, use of volunteer faculty can promote goodwill with the community at large, while involvement of emeriti faculty can ease the separation anxiety sometimes felt by new retirees.

References

1. Ness RB, Samet JM. How to be a department chair of epidemiology: a survival guide. Am J Epidemiol. 2010;172:747–51. https://doi.org/10.1093/aje/kwq268.
2. Isaac C, Lee B, Carnes M. Interventions that affect gender bias in hiring: a systematic review. Acad Med. 2009;84:1440. https://doi.org/10.1097/ACM.0b013e3181b6ba00.
3. Jacobs NN, Esquierdo-Leal J, Smith GS, Piasecki M, Houmanfar RA. Diversifying academic medicine: one search committee at a time. Front Public Health. 2022;10:854450. https://doi.org/10.3389/fpubh.2022.854450.
4. Sumra H, Riner AN, Arjani S, Tasnim S, Zope M, Reyna C, et al. Minimizing implicit bias in search committees. Am J Surg. 2022;224:1179–81. https://doi.org/10.1016/j.amjsurg.2022.05.014.
5. Kubiat NT, Guidot DM, Trim RF, Kamen DL, Roman J. Recruitment and retention in academic medicine—what junior faculty and trainees want department chairs to know. Am J Med Sci. 2012;344:24–7. https://doi.org/10.1097/MAJ.0b013e318258f205.

Chapter 18
Faculty Career Development and Wellness

Resources for Career Development

"Where Can I Find Programs That Can Help the Career Development of My Faculty?"

Most AHCs/AMCs and universities have programs to help with faculty development that can be accessed on an individual or departmental basis. Many institutions and departments also have formal career development programs for junior faculty to improve their ability to write manuscripts, prepare grant applications, create an academic advancement file, negotiate for salary and resources, etc. Additionally, several professional organizations have career development programs, some of which are tailored to specific faculty, such as Executive Leadership in Academic Medicine (ELAM) for women faculty [1], and discipline-specific resources (e.g., Association of Pathology Chairs; Alliance for Academic Internal Medicine) [2, 3]. Most business schools also have executive education courses that can help faculty develop and improve their performance in various areas (e.g., communication, negotiation, finance, management, leadership), and many companies also provide programs on these subjects.

F. Sanfilippo et al., *Lead, Inspire, Thrive*, https://doi.org/10.1007/978-3-031-41177-9_18

Implementing Career Development Programs

"How Can I Set Up an Effective Department-Wide Career Development Program?"

You should consider assigning all junior faculty appointees at least two advisors/ mentors at the time of recruitment: one in the discipline of the new faculty member to provide career counseling and guidance on professional development, and the other to oversee the general academic advancement of the new faculty member. While these advisors/mentors can be from your department, they also could be from other departments throughout your AHC/AMC and university, especially to enhance the development of interdisciplinary collaborative activities (see Chap. 29, section "Developing Joint Programs"). Having several advisors/mentors (a mentoring team) can be helpful in providing a variety of viewpoints and also reduces the possibility of conflict of interest on the part of the primary advisor/mentor [4].

Effective career development programs should be flexible and based upon the needs of the faculty member with the goal of promoting their career success [5]. It is important that the appointed advisors/mentors be compatible with their faculty member, see their potential, and be interested in helping them reach it [6]. You should require appropriate and timely feedback from faculty and their advisors/ mentors, and use it in your evaluation of the progress and performance of both.

You also may want to consider creating a leadership position (such as a vice chair for faculty affairs) to help launch and maintain career development and wellness efforts throughout your department. In addition, most institutions have experienced HR services that can be of assistance in these activities. The associate dean for faculty affairs or equivalent can be an additional useful resource, along with the support services available at your health system for clinical faculty.

Expanding Faculty Productivity

"How Can I Help Faculty Increase Their Productivity?"

In addition to providing advisors/mentors to help faculty develop their careers and increase their productivity, offering rewards and recognition can be of great benefit (see Chaps. 13 and 19). As discussed in Chap. 8, extending a faculty member's activity beyond their primary mission area(s) can be of significant benefit to them and the department. Incentivizing faculty to become more involved in those mission areas in which they are less involved can be effective in expanding collaborative activities among your clinical, research, and teaching faculty. Successful implementation of such incentives requires development and application of metrics with careful monitoring of outcomes.

You also can help faculty increase productivity by providing personal advice and suggesting that they focus on the areas in which they excel and that they enjoy the most. Interestingly, in many cases faculty are not confident about where they excel or have the greatest potential, so your advice can be very beneficial. In addition, you should consider using your contacts and influence to bring opportunities to faculty that expand their collaborations and activities, increase options for presenting their work at meetings, and provide access to important committee assignments, all of which can enhance their recognition and lead to new activities.

Depending on your institutional policies, providing time for sabbaticals can be of great value in expanding the professional interests and expertise of your faculty, refresh their career interests, enhance their wellness, and increase opportunities. Explaining the value of sabbaticals to your faculty and identifying potential sabbatical options can help them in deciding. However, always remember that the advice you give to members of your department may be mistaken as a command and potentially engender resentment. How you provide advice is as important as what advice you provide.

"How Do I Determine the Proper Use of Virtual and Remote Work for Faculty?"

Although working remotely began to develop over a decade ago, the rapid advancement of telecommunication technology and the impact of the COVID pandemic have greatly accelerated its application and use, especially for many administrative, educational, and clinical activities. An ongoing issue for remote work has been around productivity, cost, and impact, as well as the satisfaction of remote workers and those being served. Be sure to assess these factors and get input from all involved, including institutional leaders, as you develop appropriate departmental policies and individual practices for remote work.

For many administrative functions there are often cost savings with no detriment in productivity for remote work. In education, diminished personal contact has been a trade-off for expanded and easier access, and in health care there has been a sharp increase in acceptance and desire for telehealth services by consumers. As use of remote work evolves, you should be sure that agreements for splitting virtual and in-person work are explicit and in writing with any impact on compensation and benefits being completely transparent to all involved parties. Furthermore, you should ensure that the use of remote work is equitable across the faculty, and that their productivity is not sacrificed by working remotely.

Enhancing Wellness

"What Are Best Practices in Implementing a Faculty Wellness Program?"

Most institutions have wellness programs and officers who can provide consultation in setting up offerings for your department. Burnout and decreased work-life satisfaction of faculty is a major and growing problem that has been exacerbated by the recent COVID pandemic [7]. This readily spills over to staff and trainees, resulting in stress, anxiety, insomnia, depression, disengagement (so-called quiet quitting), and even suicide. It also is a major cause of medical errors, added expenses, and lost revenue [8]. While the incidence of physician burnout varies substantially by specialty, all are significantly affected, and you should be vigilant in recognizing it in your faculty and committed to creating a culture of wellness in your department.

Effective strategies for mitigating burnout and enhancing resilience for physicians have been published [9, 10] and include reducing workload through work redesign, providing counseling services, focusing on employee recognition, creating co-worker support groups, offering meditation programs, implementing time-management strategies, and creating on-the-job physical exercise programs [11]. Social functions are also important (see Chap. 11, section "Meetings and Events"), especially around graduation, holidays, and other milestone events [12].

Additional strategies include providing flexibility in work hours and remote work (see above); relaxing administrative documentation requirements whenever possible [13]; creating an equitable and inclusive working environment (see Chap. 7); providing sabbaticals (see above); streamlining software platforms to facilitate ease of use [14]; having clear standards for promotion and academic advancement; and marketing the department and its faculty and programs [12].

It is well recognized that major contributors to wellness for members of an organization are its culture and leadership behavior. There are many ways you personally can help promote wellness in your department [15], such as by:

- Explaining and communicating often about departmental goals, vision, and strategy.
- Creating strong support systems to help faculty and staff define and achieve their personal goals.
- Providing individualized expectations of roles, responsibilities, and performance.
- Engaging faculty and staff in planning and decision-making.
- Avoiding criticism of faculty and staff in any public setting.
- Signifying that well-intentioned, well-informed mistakes are welcomed and provide learning experiences.
- Bringing your department together with regularly recurring faculty meetings, town halls, retreats, and social gatherings.
- Being visible, accessible, and transparent with an open-door policy.

- Listening carefully.
- Keeping your word and commitments.
- Interacting with humility and empathy, not intimidation or arrogance.

Reviewing Performance

"What Are Best Practices in Conducting Faculty Reviews?"

Just as it is important for you to be reviewed (see Chap. 35), your faculty must be reviewed on a routine basis. Ideally this should be done annually either by you or a surrogate on your behalf (e.g., vice chairs, division chiefs, section heads). There are several ways to conduct your faculty reviews, which can differ depending on the situation. However, regular faculty reviews should involve discussion of at least the following:

- Performance over the past year relative to expectations.
- Plans and expectations for the coming year.
- Personal strengths and weaknesses.
- Potential problems and opportunities.
- Work-life balance and social well-being.
- Career development; likes and dislikes.

The time spent on each of these and other topics should be highly personalized and driven in part by the individual's priorities. Some reviews may be focused on ongoing problems that need resolution (see Chap. 20) or providing detailed advice on a specific issue or opportunity (e.g., promotion, retention, resource needs, health or personal issues). It also is useful to use the opportunity during faculty reviews to solicit candid feedback on the priorities, culture, resources, and performance of the department, as well as the performance of their supervisors, support staff, and members of your leadership team.

The review process in your department should be clearly defined, consistent with institutional procedures, and well-understood by the faculty, who should have been engaged in its development. Prior to review, faculty members should submit to you (and your surrogate reviewer if used) a written self-assessment including a summary of their accomplishments, their performance relative to expectations, and items they wish to discuss in detail. You (or your surrogate reviewer) should take written notes during or immediately after the meeting to document the discussion, evaluation, recommendations, expectations, and any disagreements.

Following the review meeting, a draft summary should be written that focuses on the evaluation and expectations set for the next review cycle, which should be reviewed and agreed to by you and the faculty member. These summaries are usually drafted by the reviewer and sent to the faculty member to respond in writing. An alternative approach is to have the faculty member draft the summary for editing by you (and your surrogate reviewer if one is used). This will engage the faculty member in their review and help ensure that they understand the summary and especially the expectations. In either case the final review letter from you (and your surrogate reviewer if used) to the faculty member should be acknowledged and agreed on in writing.

"What Are Problems That Can Occur with Reviews, and How Should I Deal with Them?"

In cases where there are disagreements, especially about past performance or proposed expectations for the following cycle, a follow-up meeting is usually necessary. If the initial review meeting was with a surrogate reviewer, the follow-up should include both of you to minimize misunderstandings and demonstrate support for your departmental leadership team. Before the follow-up meeting, the faculty member should provide documentation supporting their perspective on the issue under discussion. In cases where there is perceived noncompliance with remediation for significant problems, you should follow the procedures outlined in Chap. 20.

Since the review process should be the basis for determining changes in compensation as well as potential incentives and rewards as specified in your compensation plan (see Chap. 19), disagreements on performance or expectation may focus on the size and types of benefits being provided. To avoid these conflicts, it is important to have explicit criteria in your compensation plan that can be quantified in your review process.

Some members of your department may have a closer professional relationship to you than others (e.g., a former student or trainee, an active member of your research lab or clinical service). In such cases, conflict of interest concerns may require you to have surrogates provide the review, draft the written evaluation, and potentially co-sign the final review letter. Of course, this should not diminish your role as an advisor or mentor to such faculty in your department. However, you should be fully transparent with your leadership team about these relationships and follow their recommendations on how to proceed. Remember, especially for leaders, even the appearance of a conflict of interest needs to be managed appropriately (see Chap. 33, section "Handling Conflicts of Interest").

References

1. Executive Leadership in Academic Medicine for women faculty (ELAM). https://drexel.edu/medicine/academics/womens-health-and-leadership/elam. Accessed 17 Mar 2023.
2. Alliance for Academic Internal Medicine: Wellness and resiliency. https://www.im.org/resources/wellness-resiliency. Accessed 10 Oct 2022.

3. Sanfilippo F, Markwood P, Bailey DN. Retaining the value of former department chairs: the association of pathology chairs experience. Acad Pathol. 2020;7:2374289520981685. https://doi.org/10.1177/2374289520981685.

4. Ness RB, Samet JM. How to be a department chair of epidemiology: a survival guide. Am J Epidemiol. 2010;172:747–51. https://doi.org/10.1093/aje/kwq268.

5. Al-Jewair T, Herbert AK, Leggitt VL, Ware TL, Hogge M, Senior C, et al. Evaluation of faculty mentoring practices in seven US dental schools. J Dent Educ. 2019;83:1392–401. https://doi.org/10.21815/JDE.019.136.

6. Burgess A, van Diggele C, Mellis C. Mentorship in the health professions: a review. Clin Teach. 2018;15:197–202. https://doi.org/10.1111/tct.12756.

7. Shanafelt TD, West CP, Sinsky C, Wang H, Carlasare LE, Sinsky C. Changes in burnout and satisfaction with work-life integration in physicians during the first 2 years of the COVID-19 pandemic. Mayo Clin Proc. 2022;97:2248–58. https://doi.org/10.1016/j.mayocp.2022.09.002.

8. Shanafelt TD, Boone S, Tan L, Dyrbye LN, Sotile W, Satele D, et al. Burnout and satisfaction with work-life balance among US physicians relative to the general US population. Arch Intern Med. 2012;172:1377–85. https://doi.org/10.1001/archinternmed.2012.3199.

9. National Academies of Science, Engineering, and Medicine. Taking action against clinician burnout: a systems approach to professional well-being. Washington, DC: The National Academies Press; 2020. https://doi.org/10.17226/25521. Accessed 17 Mar 17 2023.

10. Shanafelt TD, Noseworthy JH. Executive leadership and physician Well-being: nine organizational strategies to promote engagement and reduce burnout. Mayo Clin Proc. 2013;92:129–46. https://doi.org/10.1016/j.mayocp.2016.10.004.

11. Edu-Valsania S, Laguia A, Moriano JA. Burnout: a review of theory and measurement. Int J Environ Res Public Health. 2022;19:1780. https://doi.org/10.3390/ijerph19031780.

12. Winstead DK. Advice for chairs of academic departments of psychiatry: the "ten commandments". Acad Psychiatry. 2006;30:298–300. https://doi.org/10.1176/appi.ap.30.4.298.

13. Epstein RM, Privitera MR. Finding our way out of burnout. J Oncol Pract. 2021;17:375–7. https://doi.org/10.1200/OP.21.00233.

14. Darbishire P, Isaacs AN, Miller ML. Faculty burnout in pharmacy education. Am J Pharm Educ. 2020;84:881–3. https://doi.org/10.5688/ajpe7925.

15. Bailey DN, Lipscomb MF, Gorstein F, Wilkinson D, Sanfilippo F. Life after being a pathology department chair II: lessons learned. Acad Pathol. 2017;4:2374289517733734. https://doi.org/10.1177/2374289517733734.

Chapter 19
Faculty Compensation Plans

Characteristics

"How Do I Ensure That Our Departmental Compensation Plan Is Equitable for Faculty Based on Their Activities and Performance?"

The first step in evaluating your departmental compensation plan is to determine the level of satisfaction across the department, with particular attention to those who are not satisfied with the plan. Inequitable plans typically will be perceived by some (favored) faculty as very satisfactory and in no need of change, while leaving other faculty members feeling undervalued, disillusioned, and resentful. An equitable plan usually demonstrates a level of satisfaction that is relatively homogeneous.

Financial compensation usually has several components including base salary (using standard metrics), market adjustment (based on roles and responsibilities), and incentive bonus (performance-driven). In the case of clinical faculty, additional compensation outside your department may also be provided through a separate practice plan or hospital system. Some adjunct/volunteer faculty with clinical privileges may also receive compensation from the practice plan, hospital, or your department.

The base salary level of most faculty positions is set by the institution(s) considering rank, title, workload, and years in the position. Market adjustments normally are developed by the department for the specific roles and responsibilities of the individual. Differences in faculty specialties and expertise, along with departmental leadership roles, provide distinctive market value, which must be considered for successful recruitment and retention (see Chap. 17).

Fortunately, regional and national references for most faculty salaries are available from several commercial sources and professional societies. Nevertheless,

F. Sanfilippo et al., *Lead, Inspire, Thrive*, https://doi.org/10.1007/978-3-031-41177-9_19

differences in compensation based on market adjustments can create significant tension and dissatisfaction among groups in the department, especially between those predominantly involved in clinical versus research and teaching activities. Of course, it should be understood that differences in compensation by gender and underrepresented group status are not only illegal but are also harmful to faculty productivity and morale.

Compensation plans may include additional non-salary components such as perquisites (e.g., parking, tickets to events, paid memberships), activity support (e.g., equipment, staff assistants), and nonfinancial rewards (e.g., titles, recognition). Many departments also provide an annual discretionary fund to each faculty member that is a fixed amount for everyone or distributed by rank or years of service. These often vary year to year based on the available resources of the department. Such funds, even when relatively small, can provide faculty with a positive sense of support by the department for their career development. In some cases, funds may be committed to add programmatic support for the clinical, research, teaching, outreach, or administrative activities of the faculty member, or simply to defray expenses such as for parking, meetings, and career development activities [1].

Regardless of the apparent success of your compensation plan, it is important to review it annually during your budget process and as part of updating your strategic plan. In evaluating, modifying, or developing your compensation plan, the initial steps should be developed with your leadership team, and, at the appropriate point, it is critical to be transparent and engage all the faculty members in your department and appropriate institutional leaders. You should consider much of the process as a means of educating your faculty on the parameters that might be considered (see above). The key question is how much of the department's resources should be allocated to compensation versus other priorities, the answer to which should be guided by your strategic plan (see Chap. 12).

One example of an objective formula in setting faculty salaries is described by Burns et al., who advocate that all clinical and basic science medical school departments should have a transparent compensation plan that provides faculty with options for impacting their total compensation, and should offer a minimum level of Association of American Medical Colleges (AAMC) 25th percentile with overall average compensation at the AAMC median [2].

Incentives and Bonuses

"What Activities Should I Include in an Incentive Plan?"

Incentives are usually based upon achievement of clearly defined goals. As potentially the most contentious part of your compensation plan, the specific components and relative values of incentives and financial rewards should have extensive input from faculty and institutional leadership. In some cases, personal incentives are linked to achievement of their unit with respect to departmental and institutional goals. They also might be calculated as a percent of an overall pool. The percent of total compensation provided by incentive or bonus can vary dramatically, especially for clinical faculty, where a significant component of their compensation is tied to their clinical workload [3].

For clinical service, incentive/bonus compensation indicators might include turnaround time, quality outcomes, patient and provider satisfaction surveys, RVU generation, workload, and service awards. For research they might include grant support, number of publications, citations, invited talks, and other evidence of scholarly productivity [4]. For teaching they might include student evaluations, new course development, awards, and publications on education-related research or innovation [5]. For public service, they might include committee work, mentorship, outreach programs, and local, regional, and national leadership roles. Although controversial and harder to quantify, citizenship, collegiality, and collaboration are sometimes included as part of an incentive plan (see Chap. 8).

Quantitative metrics should be established for each parameter identified in the incentive/bonus plan and endorsed by all the faculty. Occasionally, a faculty member may wish to negotiate a lower percent of incentive compensation with a higher amount of guaranteed salary to reduce their risk to total income. The reciprocal is also true if a faculty member wishes to take a higher potential incentive bonus against a lower guaranteed salary to potentially increase their total compensation. When modifying or developing a new plan, it is often best to get a consultant (internal or external to the institution) to help calculate effort and productivity metrics objectively.

Review Process

"How Should I Evaluate Performance and Productivity to Determine Appropriate Compensation?"

Each faculty member of your department should have a formal and detailed annual review, consistent with departmental and institutional policy and practice (see Chap. 18, section "Reviewing Performance"). You should personally conduct reviews of your direct reports, your leadership team, and, depending on the size of your department, as many faculty as reasonable. Each review should be based on explicit expectations made during the previous review, with assessment of performance using the agreed-upon metrics. During each review, the expectations for the following year should be discussed with agreed-upon measures, especially regarding incentive bonus payments. When disagreements arise regarding expectations and compensation, apply negotiating principles (see Chap. 10).

"How Should I Deal with Compensation for Clinical Faculty Who Want to Maintain Their High Salary but Reduce Their Clinical Load to Get a Grant or Pursue More Academic Activities?"

It is worth the time to fully explain to faculty the current market differences among different clinical specialties and research disciplines, and that changes in their effort will impact their roles and responsibilities and therefore compensation. However, to enhance collaboration and alignment across missions (see Chaps. 8 and 15, section "Alignment of Missions"), you should recognize and provide appropriate added market value in compensation for faculty who can significantly span both clinical and research expertise and productivity. The incentive/bonus plan provides an additional means to provide compensation to help adjust changes in activity for productive faculty.

"How Should I Deal with Compensation for a Research Faculty Member Who Receives or Loses a Significant Grant?"

The benefits for receiving a grant that significantly exceeds expectations should be clear and explicit in the incentive/bonus component of your compensation plan. This may include special recognition, awards, and financial bonuses. Some departments have used arrangements to provide faculty a percentage of the indirect cost recovery of a grant, although this can create potential problems in handling expectations and compensation of other revenue-generating faculty, as well as conflicts with some funding agencies. Be sure to check with your appropriate institutional leaders before providing such incentives.

When a significant grant is unexpectedly lost, a transition period of continued support may be considered, especially if the individual has had a good record of achievement. In such cases, expectations should be carefully discussed and clearly documented. Many institutions have bridge funding programs to help such individuals, and you should consider the advantages and disadvantages of developing such a bridge funding program for your department during your budget and strategic planning processes.

"How Should I Deal with Compensation for a Faculty Member Who Is No Longer Productive?"

Handling compensation for nonproductive faculty should be an explicit part of your compensation plan with clear guidelines. In most cases, the ultimate consequence for consistently not meeting expectations should be significant (i.e., reassignment, significant salary reduction, and dismissal). A potential alternative is to negotiate reduced expectations in parallel with reduced compensation and resources (e.g., space, staff support; see Chap. 10). Many institutions have developed policies for salary reduction and dismissal of nonproductive faculty including those with tenure. In most institutions, tenure is technically the protection of a faculty member's academic appointment, and not a guarantee of their compensation.

In cases where an individual has genuinely attempted to be productive, due consideration and help should be extended to improve performance or to find a more appropriate position (see Chap. 18). In cases where the individual has simply given up trying to be productive and resists appropriate expectations, the approaches described for dealing with difficult faculty are warranted (see Chap. 20).

References

1. Bailey DN, Lipscomb MF, Gorstein F, Wilkinson D, Sanfilippo F. Life after being a pathology department chair II: lessons learned. Acad Pathol. 2017;4:2374289517733734. https://doi.org/10.1177/2374289517733734.
2. Burns KH, Borowitz MJ, Carroll KC, Gocke CD, Hooper JE, Amukele T, et al. The evolution of earned, transparent, and quantifiable faculty salary compensation: the Johns Hopkins pathology experience. Acad Pathol. 2018;5:2374289518777463. https://doi.org/10.1177/2374289518777463.
3. Morrow JS, Gershkovich P, Sinard J. Measuring faculty effort: a quantitative approach that aligns personal and institutional goals in pathology at Yale. Acad Pathol. 2021;8:23742895211047985. https://doi.org/10.1177/23742895211047985.
4. Holmes EW, Burks TF, Dzau V, Hindery MA, Jones RF, Kaye CI, et al. Measuring contributions to the research mission of medical schools. Acad Med. 2000;75:303–13. https://doi.org/10.1097/00001888-200003000-00027.
5. Vivek N, Sutaria J, Chu E. Aligning compensation with values: educational RVU. J Hosp Med. 2023. https://shmabstracts.org/abstract/aligning-compensation-with-values-educational-rvu/. Accessed 28 Mar 2023.

Chapter 20
Dealing with Difficult Faculty

Considerations

"What Factors Should I Consider When Dealing with a Difficult Faculty Member?"

Your obligation as department chair is to help your faculty be as productive and successful as possible for their own benefit as well as that of the department and institution and should take preference over your own professional productivity [1]. Unfortunately, this becomes difficult with faculty whose actions conflict with departmental or institutional success, priorities, standards, and policies. The potentially detrimental effects of one individual's improper behavior on the department should never be underestimated. In fact, how to deal with difficult faculty was one of the most frequently asked questions in a survey of former department chairs [2].

There are different situations in which problems with a faculty member's behavior can occur or become evident, and several factors are needed to determine how to approach and best resolve each specific issue. These situations include, but are not limited to:

- Inappropriate behavior at meetings and/or in the workplace.
- Violation of departmental and/or institutional policy.
- Refusal to follow established expectations.
- Inappropriate use of departmental and/or institutional resources.
- Improper behavior with individual students, staff, or other faculty.
- Illegal activity.

Some of the factors to be considered when dealing with difficult faculty include:

- Departmental leadership position.
- Underrepresented group status (e.g., race, sexual orientation, religion, age, disabled).

F. Sanfilippo et al., *Lead, Inspire, Thrive*,
https://doi.org/10.1007/978-3-031-41177-9_20

- Tenure status.
- History of prior behavioral issues and problems.
- Health impairment (physical, mental, emotional).
- Source of the complaint (e.g., anonymous, relayed via someone else, internal versus external).
- External reporting requirements, e.g., research misconduct, illegal activity, Title IX violation.

Evaluation

"How Should I Evaluate a Problem Individual?"

You should have objective and transparent expectations of professional activity and conduct. If these standards are not being met by someone in your department, an evaluation of the problem should be initiated promptly. Determine the specifics of the situation with those involved and document all relevant information, including the impact of the transgressions on others as well as on the department's culture.

Try to understand the perspective of problem faculty and their points of view. Consider and evaluate potential behavioral and medical issues. Document all interactions with difficult faculty and be open and transparent in such interactions. Maintain internal notes about each meeting and engage appropriate departmental and institutional leaders in the evaluation process. Consult your HR department and legal counsel as needed for advice throughout the process. Above all, strictly follow institutional guidelines. You also may consider use of an ombudsperson or consultant as needed to objectively assess all sides of the issue.

Resolution

"How Should I Resolve Issues with Difficult Faculty?"

An important aspect of conflict resolution is to address issues directly, dispassionately, and objectively considering what is best overall for the organization and those it serves [3]. After evaluating and determining the severity of the problem, you should develop a range of appropriate steps for resolution. If basic standards are not met, remedial steps should be initiated promptly. For more serious issues, formal and even legal steps of recourse may be required [3]. As appropriate, offer alternatives and compromises that include written explicit expectations for performance with the consequences for noncompliance [4].

Be sure to follow institutional guidelines and document details of all meetings, including any offers, responses, agreements, and disagreements [5]. Engage at least one other departmental or institutional leader in the resolution process; in serious cases include at least one of them in all discussions with the individual [5]. In cases where an agreement cannot be reached, seek advice from institutional leadership and your HR department before making any unilateral decisions on resolution. Options such as dismissal, significant reassignments, or buy-outs should be handled in close partnership with the institution.

Mistakes

"What Are Some of the Serious Mistakes I Can Make in Dealing with Problem Faculty?"

Mistakes can result in empowering the problem faculty member, having to defend lawsuits for your own actions, and can even lead to your own dismissal. Some of the significant mistakes you should avoid include:

- Trying to be too considerate, not taking an issue seriously enough, or delaying action, each of which may be interpreted by others that you condone the behavior, are not aware of its significance, or are afraid to act.
- Not following departmental, institutional, and legal protocols and policies.
- Not documenting the issues, meetings, and interactions with the individual.
- Not seeking advice from your HR department.
- Offering a solution for a serious offense without prior approval by your institution.
- Not keeping your institutional leaders informed of significant faculty issues.

References

1. Chervenak FA, McCullough LB. The identification, management, and prevention of conflict with faculty and fellows: a practical ethical guide for department chairs and division chief. Am J Obstet Gynecol. 2007;197:572.e1–5. https://doi.org/10.1016/j.ajog.2007.09.012.
2. Bailey DN, Lipscomb MF, Gorstein F, Wilkinson D, Sanfilippo F. Life after being a pathology department chair II: lessons learned. Acad Pathol. 2017;4:2374289517733734. https://doi.org/10.1177/2374289517733734.
3. Willett CG. Reflections from a chair: leadership of a clinical department at an academic medical center. Cancer. 2015;22:3795–8. https://doi.org/10.1002/cncr.29588.
4. Crookston RK. Working with problem faculty: a 6-step guide for department chairs. Francisco, CA: Jossey-Bass; 2012. ISBN 978-1118242384.
5. Bailey DN, Cohen S, Gotlieb A, Lipscomb MF, Sanfilippo F. What advice current pathology chairs seek from former chairs. Acad Pathol. 2018;5:2374289518807397. https://doi.org/10.1177/2374289518807397.

Part V
Student and Trainee Issues

Medical schools have responsibility for training the next generation of clinicians and biomedical researchers; as such, department chairs are charged with ensuring that the education and training component of the quadripartite mission is successful. At many schools, education is the mission component that has the smallest budget. Given the time and effort demanded for the fiduciary responsibility of your department's clinical and research activities, as chair you must be vigilant in giving the attention needed to education and training in order to ensure a supportive and effective learning environment. Attracting a diverse cadre of students and trainees and creating an inclusive and high-quality educational experience are keys to help create a generation of clinicians, scientists, and educators who reflect the communities they will serve and provide them with the quality of service they need. Providing programs and resources for career development and wellness will help attract the best students and trainees, enhance their performance, and increase their engagement with the department during and after their education and training.

Chapter 21
Student and Trainee Recruitment

Attracting the Right Students and Trainees

"How Do I Interest Medical Students and Other Health Profession Students in Doing Rotations in My Department?"

Medical students and other health profession students are vital and inspiring members of the department, but because they usually rotate for short periods of time, they can be overlooked by both faculty and staff. As chair, you play a key role in prioritizing the importance of education in the department and in emphasizing the centrality of respect for these junior members of the team. Spending time with students can be a fruitful investment in the future since students who enjoy their rotations may develop interest in residency, fellowship, and even faculty opportunities in your department [1].

Some departmental rotations will be mandatory for students and these assignments are generally made by school administrators. However, elective rotations are selected by students and it behooves the chair and departmental faculty to attract the best students. Consideration should be given to having an "open house" to let students know about your department. Many departments also have had good success by creating special interest groups (SIGs) to attract students to their specialty. Providing role models, especially women and those from underrepresented groups, will help send the message that your department values an inclusive educational experience (see Chap. 7).

Chairs should work with their faculty to determine their capacity to extend teaching loads for trainees from other health profession programs in their AHC/AMC, providing the opportunity for multidisciplinary learning venues. In addition, the feasibility of attracting students from other institutions to do rotations in your department should be considered since this often is an effective way of recruiting future residents who are known entities to the department.

F. Sanfilippo et al., *Lead, Inspire, Thrive*, https://doi.org/10.1007/978-3-031-41177-9_21

"How Do I Attract and Recruit the Best Residents and Fellows to My Department?"

For many clinical departments, residents are essential to the effective delivery of patient care, stimulate scholarly activities, and contribute to the academic reputation of the unit. As chair you should proactively partner with faculty and staff to convince talented candidates to rank your departmental programs highly [2]. New approaches such as a shift toward digital recruitment may suggest the need for revision of recruitment materials [3].

Residents and fellows will quickly intuit the culture of your department during their interview visits, so you have the opportunity to set the tone. A warm welcome from you and some one-on-one time during their visits can go a long way in attracting the best trainees. Interview agendas should be carefully crafted and when possible tailored to the interests of the candidate. Candidate interactions with current residents and fellows, as well as select faculty and staff, are central to successful recruitments.

Highlighting the diversity of your department and providing opportunities for women and those from underrepresented groups to meet with faculty and current trainees who share their life experiences signals that your department values equity (see Chap. 7). A combination of individual chats, group gatherings, and observation of clinical and research activities should be included in the applicants' visit itineraries. You should emphasize to all members of your department, especially those who meet and interview applicants, that these visits paint a picture of your department which will be disseminated nationally as candidates return to their current institutions.

In many departments, the chair is responsible for oversight of the recruitment of house staff, usually in conjunction with the GME office and the Designated Institutional Official (DIO). You (and/or your delegate, e.g., vice chair of education) should interact with the education deans and DIO as needed to understand how residents are allocated to departments within your school and how financial responsibility is assigned. A good working relationship with these other leaders will play a major role in defining the success of your department's training programs.

"How Do I Support Faculty to Be Competitive for Attracting MS and PhD Students, as well as Post-doctoral Scholars in My Department?"

In many clinical and basic science departments, master's and PhD students are major contributors to the research, scholarly success, and reputation of the school. Science program leaders in other parts of your AHC/AMC and across the broader university are usually looking for good research opportunities for their trainees. You should take the time to meet with the leaders of graduate training programs to discuss the research training offered by your faculty, learn about the graduate school programs, and encourage your faculty to participate as members of the university's graduate schools and training grants.

Nationally, post-doctoral positions may vary highly in quality and oversight, and much has been written about prolonged, underpaid labor extracted from these scholars. Yet, post-docs can make or break faculty research success and are important training grounds for future faculty. You can avoid problems by discussing the expectations for post-docs with faculty members in whose labs such scholars are working. Increasingly, post-doctoral scholars are forming unions and advocating for increased salaries, better working conditions, and more opportunities for career development. Many perceive that options in industry are preferable to academia since faculty positions may be very limited even after they complete prolonged post-doctoral stints. Both you and faculty members should be well versed in school and university regulations about these positions, especially if trainees are unionized (see "Providing Compensation and Benefits" below), and ensure that your departmental policies and practices align with these requirements.

Providing a High-Quality Learning Environment

"What Is My Role as Chair in Helping to Shape the Curriculum for Students?"

As chair, you should ensure that your departmental faculty are continuously assessing and improving the curriculum provided to the students at your institution. Depending upon the size of your department, you may delegate responsibility for guiding curriculum development to a vice chair or expert teacher, or you may elect to do this yourself. Regardless, your department should work closely with the school educational leadership and course directors to ensure that your part of the curriculum aligns with the overall course objectives.

As part of regularly scheduled meetings, student feedback and evaluations of departmental teaching should be shared with the faculty and used as a catalyst for discussions on needed improvements. As pedagogy evolves, the classic lecture from the podium repeated and updated year-after-year has been replaced with innovations such as flipped classrooms and small group learning sessions [4]. Likewise, the increased application of AI-based technology and virtual simulation is providing alternative means of education and training that can improve competency [5]. Providing faculty with skills in these new approaches is important to ensure good learning. Quality of teaching should be an explicit part of all faculty evaluations.

Multidisciplinary training experiences are now recognized as important to prepare students and trainees to work well in teams in their future jobs [6]. As part of strategic planning and curriculum development, your department can consider ways to collaborate with other training programs to bring together student and trainee groups with diverse backgrounds.

"How Do I Ensure that Residents and Fellows Receive Effective Training in My Department?"

Training residents and fellows is a major goal in most medical school departments. Traditional "sink or swim" apprenticeship GME models are no longer acceptable and your focus should be on ensuring that trainees thrive in a supportive learning environment. As required by the Accreditation Council for Graduate Medical Education (ACGME) and other accreditation bodies, residency and fellowship should be about education, rather than service provision. If trainees are treated as a cheap source of labor, you will quickly find it difficult to attract quality candidates and the academic culture of the department will deteriorate.

As department chair, you should proactively define how much direct responsibility you will assume for the residency program and how much you want to delegate to a designated faculty member. Maintaining close interactions with the GME director, the institution's DIO, and other residency leaders is essential. Specific didactic curriculum and clinical experiences should be well-defined, with mechanisms for fair and equitable evaluations enforced. Familiarity with ACGME requirements and active participation of departmental faculty and staff, as well as trainees, in the ACGME accreditation process are essential.

Challenges can arise when residents and fellows have rotations at multiple hospitals or other clinical settings—some of which may be staffed by physicians who are not full-time faculty in your department. As department chair, you and your education leaders should be familiar with all the training venues to which your residents are assigned; ensuring comparable and high-quality experiences in each setting is essential.

"How Much Influence Should I Have on the Experience of MS and PhD Students and Post-doctoral Researchers?"

Too often master's and PhD students and post-doctoral research fellows are the forgotten trainees in the department. Unless your department has a graduate student degree program, your faculty may view the responsibility for MS and PhD students as belonging to the graduate program directors outside your department, and responsibility for the post-doctoral fellows to their individual research laboratory supervisor. These students and trainees can make many contributions to the scholarly activity and atmosphere in the department. As chair, ensuring that fair and equitable evaluation procedures are in place, and that faculty practices are consistent and supportive, can avoid issues and elevate the academic reputation of your department.

"How Can I Promote Diversity and Inclusion in the Learning Environment for Students and Trainees in My Department?"

Promoting diversity and inclusion in the learning environment is both a responsibility and an opportunity for you as chair to enhance your departmental culture (see Chap. 7). DEI starts with the choice of students and trainees; by ensuring holistic approaches in your selection processes, your department can benefit from broader perspectives among the trainee cohort [7].

You should also ensure that faculty review the curriculum to ensure that exposure to diverse patient groups, communities, and medical issues is included both in the didactic curriculum and in the clinical and research rotations. By including explicit questions about DEI in evaluations by students and trainees, your department can gauge progress in advancing these goals.

"What Should I Do if Students or Trainees Want to Lodge Concerns or Complaints About Their Experience in My Department?"

Inevitably, a student or trainee will have a negative experience and want to approach you with a concern or complaint. Before this happens, you should be sure to be aware of the institutional procedures and resources available to you and your department for responding to these issues. It behooves you to understand the policies for addressing student complaints and to know who in the dean's office and student affairs is assigned responsibility. Similarly, residency programs have defined expectations and assigned personnel for handling their complaints. When responding to serious allegations or clinical errors, it is advisable to involve and consult with the institution's legal and risk management officers.

When a student or trainee approaches you, do not dismiss or minimize their concerns. At the same time, be cautious in expressing a judgment or decision. Usually, the best course of action is to inform them of their options and then involve the appropriate school or hospital officials in developing a plan to investigate and respond. Be caring, but know that complex interpersonal interactions need to be carefully managed—avoid snap judgments!

"How Can I Optimize CME Programs Offered by My Departmental Faculty?"

CME programs offer an opportunity to highlight the expertise of your faculty and to provide service by educating providers in your community and beyond. Engaging your faculty in these courses is part of your job as chair. You should encourage discussion of whether to include CME as a goal in your department's strategic plan. If the department elects to pursue this, work closely with your CME office, show up at the sessions (your visibility sends a powerful message), and carefully review the evaluations with your faculty to identify ways to regularly improve your offerings.

Providing Compensation and Benefits

"How Are Salaries for Trainees Set? How Do I Ensure that the Pay Is Reasonable?

Salaries for residents and clinical fellows are generally set by the hospital or AHC/AMC, while PhD stipends are often prescribed by the graduate program. In contrast, compensation for research and post-doctoral fellows is more likely to be managed by the department or the medical school. Post-doctoral stipends in particular have recently garnered more attention as these scholars have begun to negotiate and unionize at some US institutions (see above). Indeed, the combination of low salaries and extended training time for many of these individuals is currently resulting in a national decline in applicants interested in these positions. Paying a living wage to trainees is a responsibility that should be embraced by you and your department and communicated to your faculty [8].

Beyond salaries, benefits for trainees may vary significantly. Chairs should understand and be supportive of sick leave and parental leave policies in their departments. Smaller perks such as access to fitness facilities can build significant goodwill with trainees. Policies on subjects such as meals provided during clinical rotations and travel stipends to attend conferences should be included in your reviews of the benefits available to trainees. Conferring with chairs of other departments at your institution and your peers at other schools can give insights about appropriate policies, standard practices, and desirable benefit levels.

As advised for faculty compensation, regular reviews of trainee salaries and benefits using institutional and national benchmarks can give valuable information about the competitiveness of the offerings in your department. You should pay specific attention to equity by gender, race, ethnicity, and other categories during these reviews.

"What Is My Role in Overseeing the Compensation Received by Post-doctoral Scholars in My Department?"

Post-doctoral researchers' salaries are often determined, at least in part, by the individual faculty member and largely on the basis of their grant funding. You should remember to review these decisions with faculty during their annual evaluation. As mentioned above, low salaries have prompted unionization at some schools; proactive decisions to provide fair compensation can help avoid confrontational approaches and promote a positive environment in your department.

References

1. Cruess SR, Cruess RL, Steinert Y. Supporting the development of a professional identify: general principles. Med Teach. 2019;41:641–9. https://doi.org/10.1080/0142159X.2018.1536260.
2. Phitayakorn R, Macklin EA, Goldsmith J, Weinstein D. Applicants' self-reported priorities in selecting a residency program. J Grad Med Educ. 2015;7:21–6. https://doi.org/10.4300/JGME-D-14-00142.1.
3. Haas MRC, He S, Sternberg K, Jordan J, Deiorio N, Chan TM, et al. Reimagining residency selection: part 1—a practical guide to recruitment in the post-covid 19 era. J Grad Med Educ. 2020;12:539–44. https://doi.org/10.4300/JGME-D-20-00907.1.
4. Hew KF, Lo CK. Flipped classroom improves student learning in health professions education: a meta-analysis. BMC Med Educ. 2018;18:38. https://doi.org/10.1186/s12909-018-1144-z.
5. Dekhtyar M, Park YS, Kalinyak J, Chudgar SM, Fedoriw KB, Johnson KJ, et al. Use of a structured approach and virtual simulation practice to improve diagnostic reasoning. Diagnosis. 2022;9:69–76. https://doi.org/10.1515/dx-2020-0160.
6. Lerner S, Magrane D, Friedman E. Teaching teamwork in medical education. Mt Sinai J Med. 2009;76:318–29. https://doi.org/10.1002/msj.20129.
7. Association of American Medical Colleges: Best practices for recruitment and retention of a diverse student body webinar 2016. https://www.aamc.org/professional-development/affinity-groups/gsa/webinars/diverse-student-recruitment. Accessed 27 Dec 2022.
8. Pasha AS, Shabeeb RA. Do differences in internal medicine resident salaries correlate with variation in cost of living? J Gen Intern Med. 2022;35:2508–9. https://doi.org/10.1007/s11606-019-05471-z.

Chapter 22
Student and Trainee Career Development and Wellness

Resources for Career Development

"What Programming Should My Department Provide for Students' and Trainees' Career Development?"

Providing specific programs to support the career development of students and trainees is a great way to send the message that you value the next generation of clinicians and researchers. You should encourage faculty to ensure that educational offerings include experiences beyond the basic curriculum. Courses in leadership, time management, negotiation skills, conflict resolution, wellness, and diversity, among others, are an important part of lifelong learning, and your department should discuss how to contribute in these areas.

It is essential that students and trainees receive mentoring and guidance on the next steps in their careers (e.g., applying for residency positions, fellowships, job opportunities). While your faculty members serve as role models for academic careers, you may want to consider partnering to introduce students and trainees to leaders in industry, government, and other arenas in your field. These types of educational experiences often are a driving force in determining which departments attract their students and trainees to stay in their specialty. Likewise, developing programs that promote networking among students of different disciplines, especially in presenting their interests and activities, can help them broaden career goals and opportunities for collaboration [1].

F. Sanfilippo et al., *Lead, Inspire, Thrive*, https://doi.org/10.1007/978-3-031-41177-9_22

"How Can I Shape the Student and Trainee Experience in My Department in a Way That Attracts Them to Our Specialty or Institution upon Graduation?"

In addition to the formal training described above, personal outreach often is the most impactful in encouraging students and trainees to choose your field for their careers or to remain at your institution (and in your department) after they complete their training. Rewarding faculty for mentoring and advising students and trainees can augment the message that your specialty and department is one in which the junior colleagues are valued—and will be valued going forward. Time, energy, and caring at this stage can be much more effective in identifying and attracting future faculty candidates than costly and time-consuming searches later.

Enhancing Achievement

"What Is My Role as Chair in the Development and Delivery of the Curriculum in My Department?"

At most schools, faculty have primary responsibility for the curriculum, and you should convey the importance of this role to your department. You also should ensure that faculty are working cooperatively with course leaders along with education deans and staff at your institution. Your review and constructive questions about the curriculum can help improve the courses and training offered in your department and thus improve your department's reputation.

As discussed in Chaps. 15 and 21, you must decide how much teaching you will do as chair. Involvement in at least one student course and contributions to resident/fellow training in clinical and research settings will be noticed (and appreciated) and can set the tone for the importance of the educational mission in your department.

"What Characteristics of the Learning Environment Are Important for Achieving Student Success?"

New pedagogical approaches and education technology may necessitate additional faculty training to optimize the learning environment in your department. Further, ensuring that the departmental culture is supportive, inclusive, and free of harassment is essential (see Chap. 7). Insights can be gained from periodic reviews of student and resident evaluations of the faculty and their experiences; these can then guide the department in needed modifications or corrective actions. Discovering during an accreditation review that the learning environment in your department is poorly rated is too late—proactive assessment is key!

"How Can I Ensure That Trainees Achieve Their Full Potential Through the Experiences Offered in My Department?"

Encouraging a departmental culture in which education is valued and where students and other trainees are viewed as valuable assets will be enhanced by recognizing your faculty who excel in these activities. You should consider giving departmental awards to outstanding teachers and creating a "master educator" academy [2]. You can feature excellence in teaching in your communications, such as departmental newsletters, recognize the best educators during annual performance reviews, and reward them as part of your faculty compensation plan (see Chap. 19).

Promoting Wellness

"How Can the Department Enhance Wellness Among the Medical and Other Health Profession Students and Trainees in My Department?"

Student and trainee wellness requires ongoing attention and work [3]. Because there are inherent stresses in didactic, clinical, and research training, the physical and mental health of students and residents must be of paramount importance [4]. Recently, more attention has been extended to the post-doc experience, with high levels of stress and burnout identified [5].

Your department should have well-communicated procedures for responding to student and trainee health crises. You should be familiar with the wellness resources available to students and trainees and ensure that your faculty members know about these as well. Student and trainee orientation should include an overview of these procedures and resources.

Of course, proactive promotion of wellness is preferable to crisis management. As chair, you should communicate to faculty and staff the expectations of having a bias- and harassment-free culture in your department. Emphasizing that students and trainees will thrive in a supportive, nurturing environment is to everyone's benefit.

Most AHCs/AMCs have established student wellness programs, although they vary in the services and resources offered [6]. These may include counseling services, employee recognition, organized volunteer activities, support groups, meditation programs, gym or fitness facility access, emergency financial assistance, special training classes, and more (see Chap. 18, section "Enhancing Wellness"). Many institutions have appointed a wellness officer or leader: you (or your delegate) should work with this person to understand the available services, share information about the resources with your departmental faculty and staff, and consider creation of department-specific offerings.

"What Do I Do When a Student or Trainee Manifests a Mental Health Issue?"

Mental health challenges will undoubtedly arise for a student or trainee in your department—early identification and nonjudgmental interventions can help prevent tragic consequences. Faculty and staff should be trained in procedures and resources for responding to such crises, which should be done on a regular basis, not just after an acute problem is identified. Confidentiality is imperative and caring can make a huge difference in the outcome. Wellness resources and professional providers are likely available at your institution and should be utilized proactively.

The return to training after treatment for a mental health issue can be challenging for both the student/trainee and the rest of the department. As chair, you can set a welcoming, nonjudgmental tone and convey that the student/trainee is still a valued member of the program.

Reviewing Performance

"What Are Good Approaches for Evaluating Student and Trainee Performance in My Department?"

Faculty are primarily responsible for student and trainee evaluations, but valuable insights can also be obtained from staff, patients, and others. Standardized approaches to evaluation are important to ensure equitable assessment. Expectations and evaluation procedures should be clearly delineated to students and trainees at the onset of their experience in your department. Timely feedback is key, and delayed reports mean missed chances for effective formative evaluation and improvement. In addition, at many institutions, late clinical evaluations have been a source of concern during accreditation visits.

As chair, you should regularly analyze the evaluation processes and results for students/trainees in your department. Questions to address should include:

- Are students and trainees in your department performing adequately on shelf exams and other tests compared to national norms? This can help faculty identify areas for curriculum reform or changes in faculty teaching assignments.
- Is there comparability among faculty in how students and trainees are rated? If there are faculty who routinely give overly positive or negative reviews, you can

provide feedback to that faculty member so that students are more fairly evaluated.

- Are there any trends in student or trainee evaluations which suggest gender, racial/ethnic, or other biases? If your periodic review suggests this, it should be a focus area for discussion with faculty and other evaluators.

"How Do I Ensure That Students and Trainees Are Being Accurately and Fairly Evaluated by the Faculty in My Department?"

Periodic reviews of trends in student and trainee evaluation can provide useful insights to raise awareness in your department. Unfortunately, ongoing bias in evaluation on the basis of gender, race/ethnicity, sexual orientation, and more continues to be documented. If biases are found in your department, rapid intervention is required. Discussion at faculty meetings, including additional training of evaluators, can help attenuate bias and enhance the objectivity of evaluations.

"What Should I Do When Suboptimal Performance by a Student or Trainee Is Reported or Observed?"

While it is hoped that every student and trainee will perform well, suboptimal and even unacceptable performances will occur [7]. If individual feedback and guidance delivered by the responsible faculty member does not correct the problem, you may need to facilitate access to provide additional expertise. Discussion with educational specialists from the dean's staff or with a "master teacher" can be useful.

Clearly communicating the specific requirements for student/trainee performance to be considered satisfactory should be provided to them early and continuously. Unfortunately, especially with short-term rotations, the practice has too often been to pass the problem on. While it is more work to address issues than to hope that problems will be corrected by others down the line, providing constructive feedback is an important role for every teacher and supervisor of students and trainees. You should make it clear that this is an expected activity for faculty and provide the advice, training, and resources needed to help them improve the student/trainee's performance.

In rare instances, egregious issues may prompt the need for a student or trainee to be removed (at least temporarily while the situation is investigated) from classes and training. This is particularly true for behaviors during clinical training, such as abuse of a patient or dangerous error in clinical judgment. In such cases, close coordination with the appropriate staff in your school and hospital/clinic is essential, as well as with risk management officers and legal counsel to ensure compliance with regulatory and legal requirements.

References

1. Kumarasamy MA, Sanfilippo F. Breaking down silos: engaging students to help fix the US health care system. J Multidiscip Healthc. 2015;8:101–8. https://doi.org/10.2147/JMDH.S79384.
2. Chang A, Schwartz BS, Harleman E, Johnson M, Walter LC, Fernandez A. Guiding academic clinician educators at research-intensive institutions: a framework for chairs, chiefs, and mentors. J Gen Intern Med. 2021;36:3113–21. https://doi.org/10.1007/s11606-021-06713-9.
3. Posselt JR. Promoting graduate student Well-being: cultural, organizational and environmental factors in the academy. Washington, DC: Council of Graduate Schools; 2021. https://cgsnet.org/wp-content/uploads/2022/01/CGS_Well-being-ConsultPaper-Posselt.pdf. Accessed 20 Mar 2023.
4. Leshner AI, Scherer LA. Mental health, substance use, and wellbeing in higher education: supporting the whole student, vol. 2021. Washington, DC: The National Academies Press; 2021. https://nap.nationalacademies.org/download/26015.
5. Woolston C. Postdocs under pressure: can i even do this anymore. 2020. https://www.nature.com/articles/d41586-020-03235-y#. Accessed 27 Dec 2022.
6. Klein HJ, McCarthy SM. Student wellness trends and interventions in medical education: a narrative review. Humanit Soc Sci Commun. 2022;9:92. https://doi.org/10.1057/s41599-022-01105-8.
7. Patel RS, Tarrant C, Bonas S, Shaw RL. Medical students' personal experience of high-stakes failure: case studies using interpretative phenomenological analysis. BMC Med Educ. 2015;15:86. https://doi.org/10.1186/s12909-015-0371-9.

Chapter 23
Dealing with Difficult Students and Trainees

Considerations

"Whose Responsibility Is It to Address Student or Trainee Problems?"

In most cases, student and trainee performance issues are first dealt with by the responsible faculty member. This is often sufficient to provide the feedback needed for the trainee to correct the problem, which demonstrates the educational process in action. However, if the feedback does not have this desired effect and issues are ongoing, further intervention is needed. For students, you may wish to involve the education deans at your institution or, if available, the educational remediation/support services at the school. Working with the student's advisor allows the advisor to put the current problems in context of the student's overall performance in the program. For residents or fellows, the DIO, GME program director, or graduate school leader, as appropriate and available, should be involved. Their engagement can provide insights into whether the problem is isolated in your department or part of ongoing or broader performance issues.

As previously mentioned, some issues such as significant clinical errors or inappropriate interactions with patients will prompt involvement of others, including clinical leaders, risk management, and legal counsel. Especially in these instances, careful documentation of your actions as chair should be kept in your files; if lawsuits emanate from the situation, this documentation can help prevent problems for you and the department and ensure that a fair resolution is reached. Getting advice in dealing with student performance issues is always helpful [1–4].

F. Sanfilippo et al., *Lead, Inspire, Thrive*, https://doi.org/10.1007/978-3-031-41177-9_23

Evaluation

"What Resources Are Available for Me to Help Students/ Trainees Who Are Experiencing Difficulties in My Department?"

The good news is that increased attention is being paid to the well-being of students and trainees. You should be aware of the institutional resources that are available to support students and trainees during their educational experiences, such as those provided by your school or hospital, as well as those that can be accessed through national programs such as Ed Hub of the American Medical Association (AMA) [5].

Many schools now have dedicated mental health counselors who are available to trainees. You and your faculty should be familiar with these services and communicate the availability of them to students and trainees. In addition, education deans and the DIO for the GME program should be actively involved in supporting students and trainees who are experiencing difficulties. As chair, you should ensure that information about these resources is provided as part of the orientation process for new students and trainees in your department and is reviewed with them when problems are detected.

"What Is My Responsibility for Monitoring Trends in Student and/or Trainee Performance Difficulties in My Department?"

You should undertake periodic assessments to determine if there are any recurring issues in your department that need to be addressed. You can do this yourself or delegate the responsibility to a departmental vice chair for education or other senior leader on your leadership team.

Resolution

"What Is the Best Approach to Remedying Problems Identified in Student and Trainee Performance?"

As chair, you should emphasize to faculty the importance of early identification of student or trainee performance difficulties, appropriate and timely interventions, and options for referral to school or clinical resources. Input from education experts in the school (e.g., education support office, education deans, student or resident ombudsperson, or legal counsel) should be requested as needed to help guide development of corrective action plans.

Too often, problem students or residents/fellows are tolerated or ignored, rather than proactively identified and counseled or coached to address issues. This may result in the trainee being passed on to the next rotation even though the problematic performance has not been corrected. Unfortunately, this means missed opportunities for the student/trainee to improve and can result in the completion of their studies without attaining needed competencies. Your department has the responsibility to honestly evaluate trainees to determine that they at least meet minimum standards.

"How Do I Respond to Inquiries from Another Institution or a Potential Employer About Students/Trainees Who Have Performed Poorly or Been Disciplined?"

If the trainee was deemed to pass the course or rotation, a factual statement to that effect may be appropriate. But if the student or trainee failed or had to be disciplined, the situation is more challenging, and it is advisable to seek advice from others such as education deans, the DIO, and legal counsel before responding. Such requests should not be avoided or ignored; giving honest assessments informs others before the student or trainee is hired for a new position where the problem is likely to be rediscovered and reflect poorly on your department.

Mistakes

"To Whom and How Should I Disclose Information About Students/Trainees Who Make Clinical Errors or Violate Research Regulations?"

Substandard performance that meets minimum requirements should be distinguished from errors or violations that require regulatory or legal reporting to authorities. As mentioned earlier, you and your faculty should be informed and aware of the policies and procedures in place for reporting such issues.

If a trainee makes a significant clinical error, this should immediately be reported through the hospital or clinic mechanisms and investigated as any other patient error. Similarly, if a trainee violates research regulations (such as animal welfare concerns), this should be expeditiously reported to the appropriate institutional research officials. Allegations that student or trainees have committed acts of sexual harassment or have mistreated members of protected groups should be reported per institutional protocols, and expert HR advice should be obtained. Legal counsel and your communications staff can be very valuable in advising you about the appropriate interactions with media, regulators, or potential employers in these situations, and you should remain in touch with the status of any investigation.

References

1. Ferguson CC, Ark TK, Kalet AL. REACH: a required curriculum to foster the Well-being of medical students. Acad Med. 2022;97:1164–9. https://doi.org/10.1097/ACM.0000000000004715.
2. Moonaghi HK, Emadhadeh A, GharibNavaz R, Rad M, Sabeghi H, AshrafiFard H, et al. Challenging behaviors in medical students: clarification of observations of professors. Res Dev Med Educ. 2020;9:6. https://doi.org/10.34172/rdme.2020.006.
3. Ronan-Bentle SE, Avegno J, Hegarty CB, Manthey DE. Dealing with the difficult student in emergency medicine. Int J Emerg Med. 2011;4:39. https://doi.org/10.1186/1865-1380-4-39.
4. Yavari N, Asghari F, Shahvari Z, Nedjat S, Larijani B. Obstacles of professional behavior among medical trainees: a qualitative study from Iran (2018). J Educ Health Promot. 2018;8:193. https://doi.org/10.4103/jehp.jehp_272_19.
5. Dyrbye L. Medical student well-being—minimize burnout and improve mental health among medical students. Chicago, IL: American Medical Association; 2019. https://edhub.ama-assn.org/steps-forward/module/2757082. Accessed 27 Dec 2022.

Part VI
Staff Issues

High-quality staff members are central drivers of success for your faculty and play key roles in facilitating your work and advancing the departmental mission. Recruitment and retention of staff who enhance the culture and performance of your department are critical, as is providing an environment and resources that facilitate their productivity and promote their career development and well-being. Providing competitive compensation is key to recruiting and retaining excellent staff and should be supplemented with appropriate rewards and recognition. Regular performance reviews by supervisors should include constructive feedback on strengths and action plans to address weaknesses. Staff who are nonproductive, disruptive, or difficult can impact the culture and stability of the department if not dealt with appropriately. Serious staff mistakes, especially involving students or patients, should be addressed quickly and reported as necessary, with engagement of appropriate institutional officials to determine resolution. Your appreciation and treatment of staff will be recognized by many as behaviors to be emulated, and will have a significant impact on the performance and success of your department.

Chapter 24
Staff Recruitment and Retention

Identifying the Right People for the Jobs

"Should I Keep My Predecessor's Staff?"

Your success as a new chair will be leveraged by having high-quality staff in the department, especially those who support you and the department in day-to-day operations and in building for long-term success. If you are a new chair, you will inherit staff and you should meet with key employees early in your term to exchange ideas and share your expectations and aspirations for their contributions to the team. Most of these existing staff will bring valuable insights about the history and operations of the department and can be very useful in the transition to your new leadership role. If you find an employee who is not aligned with your vision and resistant to the change, the ideal outcome is working with them (with support from the institutional HR office) to find an alternative placement and maintain good will.

"How Do I Build My Own Team of High-Functioning Staff for My Department?"

Over time, you will be able to build your own staff team. One of the most important positions is the departmental senior administrator (Chap. 11, section "Leadership Positions") [1]. This person can make your work as chair much easier and smoother, especially as you delegate oversight of many administrative day-to-day operations. Also, your personal EA is of utmost importance in helping to organize your work life and reflect a professional culture to internal and external constituents. Both these individuals and other key staff members also can serve as helpful sounding

© The Author(s), under exclusive license to Springer Nature Switzerland AG 2023

F. Sanfilippo et al., *Lead, Inspire, Thrive*,

https://doi.org/10.1007/978-3-031-41177-9_24

boards. They also can be central to the "informal" organizational chart in your department, fielding questions and concerns that others may be reluctant to bring to you directly (see Chap. 11, section "Leadership Positions", and Chap. 36) [2]. It is well worth taking the time and effort to find the best people for these and other key positions in your department.

Staff can have a significant positive or negative impact on the reputation and performance of you and your department [3]. Soon after you become chair, you should review the organizational chart for staff in your department and ask questions that will help you understand the roles and responsibilities of key personnel:

- Are there any gaps in staffing of key areas? If so, why and how can they be addressed?
- Do staff work together in collaborative and collegial ways?
- Is there diverse representation among staff, and do staff perceive and advance an inclusive work environment (see Chap. 7)?
- How much of the operations work is done by departmental staff, and what is done by staff who report at the school or institutional level? (This may be particularly important in areas such as financial planning and accounting; HR, including hiring; support services such as IT; and clinical assignments/scheduling.)
- Are there dual reporting relationships to you and to others for key personnel? For example, do the departmental finance people report to the hospital or faculty practice plan as well as to you (see Chap. 11)?
- If there are staff with dual reporting, are expectations aligned and performance evaluation criteria jointly established (see Chap. 29)?
- Is compensation equitable and competitive? Replacing staff is costly and can be disruptive; it is usually better to nurture and retain good employees.

If you find your department's organizational chart to be appropriate, clearly articulate your endorsement of the current structure to all of those impacted. If you think changes will improve departmental operations, work closely with key departmental and institutional leaders to double-check the validity and feasibility of the changes you propose. Also, it may be worthwhile to assess the core competencies of your senior staff and consider if a realignment of their responsibilities might improve overall productivity and job satisfaction.

As discussed in Chap. 11 section "Operations and Administration"), you should understand which staff functions are managed at the departmental level and which are overseen at the level of your AHC/AMC or university. Shared services can be cost-effective and improve quality, especially for smaller units (see Chap. 13, section "People" and Chap. 29, section "Resources and Recognition") [4]. However, before proposing or agreeing to share services, you should understand the financial arrangements (e.g., recharges, etc.), supervisory control, and quality assurance mechanisms for the shared service.

Recruiting New Staff

"When Should I Recruit from Inside the Institution and When Should I Look Outside?"

When the need to recruit a new staff member is identified, you will have to decide whether to look internally or recruit from outside your department or institution. Internal candidates often have more knowledge of the operations and cultures of your department and your AHC/AMC, which can facilitate onboarding and productivity. In some cases, looking outside your department, your school, or your institution(s) may be preferable, especially if you are in the process of developing a novel program, trying to significantly change your departmental culture, or seeking talent that does not typically reside in an AHC/AMC (e.g., specialized areas of business, marketing, technology, etc.).

Establishing a relationship with your HR representative before needing to recruit can be very helpful. You should work closely with these experts in creating a job description, deciding whether to use a search firm (e.g., for very specialized or high-level positions), interviewing applicants, and selecting the best candidate. Standardized recruitment processes are key to developing a diverse pool of candidates and to finding the most qualified ones. This includes your recruitment strategy, approach to advertising (including posting in places accessed by diverse candidates), interview and selection processes, parameters for extending offers, setting of compensation levels, and plans for onboarding. Involving current departmental staff in the recruitment process can help provide insights and enhance the successful transition of the new employee into your department.

"How Can I Enhance DEI for Staff in My Department?"

As department chair, you should emphasize the importance of recruiting and supporting a diverse staff in your department (see Chap. 7). Having a diverse staff creates a welcoming environment and brings new perspectives and enhanced performance to operations in your department. Many departments have endorsed practices requiring that slates of potential candidates include representation from diverse groups, with attention to gender and race/ethnicity, as well as other personal attributes and backgrounds. You can help ensure that search committees and interview itineraries include diverse members and that search committee members have been educated about unconscious and other forms of bias [5].

You should work with your HR department to periodically review the diversity of the staff in your department and monitor DEI metrics in your department (see

Chap. 7 section "Measuring Success"). Careful listening can help you understand the varying experiences of all staff members, while compensation reviews and interventions to correct inequities send powerful messages about the culture of your department. Public recognition of accomplishments of diverse staff members also helps establish an inclusive work setting.

Instruments and benchmarks (both national and regional) for DEI are available, and the results should be shared with all departmental faculty and staff members, as well as institutional leaders. More and more institutions are evaluating pay equity, but other factors such as "non-salary compensation" (e.g., resources, recognition, career development opportunities, and sponsorships) continue to be assessed less frequently. Ensuring diversity of staff is a critical step in demonstrating your leadership and in achieving departmental excellence.

Retaining Current Staff

"What Are Tips for Keeping Talented Staff in the Department?"

Retaining talented staff helps maintain continuity and smooth operations in your department. It is also less costly and less time- and effort-consuming than hiring new employees. Formal events to recognize key staff members for their performance will be well received—it is especially effective if staff are celebrated at events that include faculty, community leaders, and donors in the audience. Don't forget to inform key institutional leaders, including the dean, hospital CEO (chief executive officer), and university leaders of these accomplishments (preferably in writing) and invite them to the event.

Small day-to-day recognitions can be the most important. Remember to say thank-you for jobs well done by your staff. Personal congratulatory or thank-you notes, especially when handwritten, are particularly impactful (see Chap. 5). And stay connected on a personal level—asking about an ailing spouse or about a grandchild's graduation makes employees feel recognized and appreciated.

In addition, taking the time to share lunch or celebrate birthdays with your staff will be noticed! A card or small gift at holiday time and bringing donuts when there is an early meeting are activities that communicate you care about your staff as people, not just as workers.

"When Should Remote Work Be Considered for Staff Members?"

Establishing a policy about remote or virtual work for staff members should be done in advance of individual negotiations. Many considerations should go into whether remote work is desirable in your department, and you should involve key faculty and staff, as well as HR personnel, institutional leaders, and (if appropriate) union representatives, in discussions about the policy.

Allowing remote work may attract potential employees, thus increasing the quality and diversity of the pool. Generational differences in expectations about remote work options are increasingly being recognized, with younger workers in particular often expecting this flexibility. On the other hand, concerns about the impact on departmental culture, communication, productivity, and cost need to be considered. Once a departmental policy has been established, attention should be paid to the equitable and transparent implementation for individual employees, and any unintended consequences that may have arisen. Productivity measures should be adopted to ensure that remote work does not negatively impact output.

References

1. Ness RB, Samet JM. How to be a department chair of epidemiology: a survival guide. Am J Epidemiol. 2010;172:747–51. https://doi.org/10.1093/aje/kwq268.
2. Wu F, Dixon-Woods M, Aveling E, Campbell A, Willars J, Tarrant C, et al. The role of the informal and formal organization in voice about concerns in healthcare: a qualitative interview study. Soc Sci Med. 2021;280:1–9. https://doi.org/10.1016/j.socscimed.2021.114050.
3. Fisher M. Being chair: a 12-step program for medical school chairs. Int J Med Educ. 2011;2:147–51. https://doi.org/10.5116/ijme.4ece.862d.
4. Schulz V, Brenner W. Characteristics of shared service centers. Transform Gov. 2010;4:210–9. https://doi.org/10.1108/17506161011065190.
5. Rosenkranz KM, Arora TK, Termuhlen PM, Stain SC, Misra S, Dent D, et al. Equity and inclusion in medicine: why it matters and how do we achieve it? J Surg Educ. 2021;78:1058–65. https://doi.org/10.1016/j.jsurg.2020.11.013.

Chapter 25
Staff Career Development and Wellness

Career Development, Succession Planning, and Training

"How Should I Support the Career Development of Key Staff Members in My Department?"

Supporting the career development of key staff members is a worthwhile investment by you and your department, which will yield a high return. You should encourage staff to take advantage of both internal training opportunities and external courses, which may range from a class on computer skills for clerical staff to attendance at professional meetings and to certificate courses and credentialing opportunities. You also should decide on an appropriate departmental budget for such training opportunities and determine how candidates for participation will be chosen. There also may be funding available through the school, hospital, university, and external corporate sponsors.

Staff are more likely to leave if they don't see a chance to advance within your department. One way to address this is by creating career ladders for key employees, which your HR department can help you develop and implement [1]. Career ladders (or "roadmaps") are designed to formally advance a staff employee to a higher level of job responsibility. Career ladders help employees see an exciting future in the department and provide the chance for them to attain their full potential without having to job-hop. This can help your department achieve fewer missed workdays, higher employee satisfaction, and improved performance overall.

Mentoring is not only for faculty and students; it is also important for staff. Assigning advisors/mentors to new staff can help in their transition and subsequent career development. You also might consider identifying one or two key staff to be personal mentors, being careful to avoid other staff believing that they are receiving special attention because they are your "favorites." In most cases, you should be

F. Sanfilippo et al., *Lead, Inspire, Thrive*,
https://doi.org/10.1007/978-3-031-41177-9_25

able to assign other staff members, either within the department or elsewhere in your AHC/AMC (or beyond), who can fill the role as staff mentors.

"What About Succession Planning for Staff?"

As for faculty, succession planning for key staff positions should be a priority. Without advance planning, operations can be seriously disrupted when a staff member unexpectedly announces that they plan to leave the department or when an emergency requires a prolonged or permanent absence. For your personal staff reports, you should identify individuals who could step in to each position on a temporary basis. You should determine if this work could be done by an existing staff member for a short period or if temporary hires will be needed to do the job or backfill the role. In addition, you should expect all supervisors to have these plans in place for other key personnel.

Routine turnover and advancement offer the opportunity to consider if other employees can be promoted to fill a position. This can be a key part of developing career ladders for your employees as described above. Alternatively, external hiring of full- or part-time staff may be needed to augment the existing staff. A good practice during an annual review of your strategic plan or budget process is to determine and document which employees could be promoted to fill key staff positions in the event of openings. Identifying candidates as "ready now," "ready in 1–2 years," or "ready in 3–5 years" can be a useful approach. For those not yet ready, the additional training or experience needed to prepare them should be clarified and pursued. This allows more predictable approaches to staffing and identifies roles that will require searching outside of the department or institution. The National Institutes of Health (NIH) has published a helpful guide for staff succession planning [2].

Enhancing Productivity

"How Can I Incentivize My Team to Be a High-Performing Group?"

Staff recognition programs can dramatically enhance departmental morale. Periodic announcements about employees who have made special contributions encourage enthusiastic effort and greater creativity. Such recognition might include "employee of the month" programs, newsletter stories, or special perks (e.g., a convenient parking space or free coffee in the staff room). Further, you should recognize great team performances in addition to individual efforts. Highlighting the work of a group on an ongoing program or a special initiative will incentivize willingness to work collaboratively as a team (see Chap. 8, section "Stimulating Collaboration" and Chap.

11, section "Building Your Team"). Of course, these recognition programs should augment, not serve as a substitute for, equitable and competitive compensation and benefits (see Chap. 26).

Periodic staff meetings are important venues for communicating information and involving staff. While these may be arranged and overseen by a key staff assistant, you should ask to be included on the agenda to provide departmental updates and to thank staff for their contributions.

Promoting Wellness

"How Can I Help Staff Thrive in My Department?"

You should make sure that staff are informed about and encouraged to use institutional wellness programs and services that your AHCs/AMCs has available for them, which may range from mental health services to meditation programs and access to gym and fitness rooms. You may also want to consider organizing an off-site staff field trip and other events that encourage staff to interact and get to know each other outside of their day-to-day work activities. A number of resources describe characteristics of effective wellness programs for staff [3–5]. The participation of key faculty leaders in these staff programs can add significant benefits for team building and your organizational culture.

Perhaps the most important way to ensure that staff thrive is by providing opportunities for authentic engagement in departmental activities. Staff should be represented in the strategic planning process, key hiring decisions, and major policy discussions (see Chap. 11, section "Building Your Team" and Chap. 12). If your employees belong to a union, you can reach out to union representatives and include them as appropriate.

Reviewing Performance

"What Are Best Practices for Reviewing the Performance of Departmental Staff?

Formal staff performance reviews should take place at an established time on an annual basis, or more frequently if prescribed by institutional policy. The best performance reviews should offer helpful advice and serve as a venue for acknowledging important contributions and should not be unexpectedly punitive or used to convey feedback that should have been provided throughout the year. Procedures should be transparent, expectations should be clearly delineated in advance, and evaluations should be equitable.

A best practice is to ask the staff member to do a written self-assessment in advance of the meeting; this can include a summary of their accomplishments over the last year and goals for the upcoming year, as well as self-identified areas for improvement. At the review meeting, these should be discussed, the supervisor's input documented, and a written summary of the discussion agreed to. As chair, you can role model these practices with reviews of your direct reports and communicate these expectations to others when they review their staff.

Lapses in performance may require formal documentation along with corrective action plans, which should be undertaken as soon as possible after the performance issue becomes apparent. Hopefully, the corrective action plan will resolve the issue and reduce the need for low ratings in the annual performance review. If not, the documentation provides important support for a negative year-end review.

In addition to the formal annual evaluation, informal reviews and feedback should be provided on a continuous basis, as formative rather than summative evaluations. Suggestions for improvement provide the opportunity for staff to add skills and increase work quality. Additionally, documentation of superior performance provides a chance to celebrate special achievements, and a letter to the staff member's file can help support promotion and salary adjustments.

"Should I Delegate Performance Reviews to Others?"

You personally should do performance reviews only for your direct reports, which should be very limited in number. Other performance reviews should be delegated to your chief administrative officer, chief of staff, and staff managers/supervisors, as appropriate.

References

1. Society for Human Resource Management: Developing employee career paths and ladders. SHRM toolkit. https://www.shrm.org/resourcesandtools/tools-and-samples/toolkits/pages/developingemployeecareerpathsandladders.aspx. Accessed 27 Dec 2022.
2. National Institutes of Health Office of Human Resources. https://hr.nih.gov/sites/default/files/public/documents/2021-03/Succession_Planning_Step_by_Step_Guide.pdf. Accessed 28 Mar 2023.
3. Jones D, Molitor D, Reif J. What do workplace wellness programs do? Evidence from the Illinois workplace wellness study. Q J Econ. 2019;134:1747–91. https://doi.org/10.1093/qje/qjz023.
4. Mattke S, Liu H, Caloveras J, Huang CY, Van Busum KR, Khodyakov D, et al. Workplace wellness programs study: final report. Rand Health Q. 2013;3:7. https://www.rand.org/pubs/research_reports/RR254.html. Accessed 28 Mar 2023.
5. Song Z, Baicker K. Effect of a workplace wellness program on employee health and economic outcomes. JAMA. 2019;321:1491–501. https://doi.org/10.1001/jama.2019.3307.

Chapter 26
Staff Compensation

Salaries and Benefits

"How Are Salaries and Benefits Set for Staff in My Department?"

As chair, you should understand how your departmental policies, standards, and practices for staff salaries and benefits were developed and currently applied. In some cases, salaries (or salary ranges) are determined system-wide at the level of the AHC/AMC, including those set by union contracts if applicable at your institution(s). However, your department may have the discretion, at least within salary ranges, to request step or merit increases, and there are published guides to assist in setting salary ranges [1]. Some employees may value salary over benefits such as retirement savings plans (especially younger employees who often do not plan to stay at the institution as long), and, as allowed by institutional policy, it may be advisable to tailor the balance of salary and benefits to the individual. Familiarity with these policies and a close working relationship with your HR colleagues will help keep salaries and benefits up to date and appropriate.

"What Do I Need to Consider if My Staff Are Represented by Unions?"

At a growing number of AHCs/AMCs, staff are now members of unions—from nurses in clinical settings to support staff and physicians. Recently, post-doctoral scholars, resident physicians, and staff clinicians have been exploring union

F. Sanfilippo et al., *Lead, Inspire, Thrive*,
https://doi.org/10.1007/978-3-031-41177-9_26

representation as a way to improve work environments and increase their compensation, and at some institutions this has already happened. You should have a clear understanding of which staff in their department (and with whom they interact across the institution) are members of unions and which unions represent department members. You and your leadership team are well advised to track proposed union stances, votes, and potential labor actions, even if you do not directly negotiate with the unions (which is usually done by institutional leaders and HR experts). For staff who are unionized, you should understand how much leeway you have when setting salaries (e.g., within ranges negotiated by the union) and what working conditions have been agreed to by the union and institution. It can be challenging when some staff are represented by unions and others are not, especially when they work "side by side" with overlapping responsibilities but have different salary structures and compensation. Whenever and however possible, it is advisable to strive for equity between the unionized and nonunionized staff in your department to avoid friction and enhance collegiality and teamwork.

"How Do I Deal with the Fact That Contracted Employees (e.g., Traveling Nurses) May Be Paid Substantially More than Staff Employees?"

Many AHCs/AMCs have turned to contract employees to fill gaps in their staffing, a phenomenon that was exacerbated during the pandemic. The most frequently cited example of this is traveling nurses who were hired as patient care needs surged and staff nurses left (or took leaves) from the institution. In many cases, these contract employees had significantly higher compensation than institutional staff, creating tensions and resentments when the work being done was comparable but the salaries were not. In such cases, (partial) equity adjustments were sometimes made for existing staff, often with budgetary strain. You should be aware of these challenges and interact closely with HR representatives to address the issues as fairly as possible when they arise.

In some cases, contract employees can be cost-effective, especially if they are needed for a defined length of time, have specialized skills, or can make contributions that improve performance and revenues. It is important to remember that high hourly rates sometimes reflect, at least in part, the fact that non-salary benefits (e.g., health insurance, etc.) may not be provided by the institution, at least to the degree enjoyed by regular full-time (and many part-time) employees.

Work Assignments

"How Do I Ensure That Expectations of Staff Are Fair and Linked Appropriately to Compensation?"

You should convey your expectation to supervisors that job assignments and work-load requirements are fairly distributed among staff. Morale can be seriously eroded if staff members perceive that others are not pulling their weight. Various tools can be helpful in making these assessments, including time-management studies.

In addition, you should assess whether your department reflects occupational segregation (i.e., bias toward filling certain positions with women or those from under-represented groups based on historical stereotypes). Further, it is important to be alert to "gender taxes" or "minority taxes" (e.g., overusing women or those from underrepresented groups for department and school/university service, see Chap. 7) [2].

"What Do I Do When Unionized Staff Go on Strike?"

In the event of a strike, it is critical for you to work closely with institutional leaders and HR representatives and to align with institutional practices. You should work with these colleagues to determine which activities are essential and must continue during the strike (e.g., critical patient service, care of research animals, etc.) and how these essential activities can be maintained. In some instances, work duties can be reallocated among non-striking staff including supervisors, but in other instances, temporary replacements may be identified if advised and approved by institutional leaders. After the strike is resolved, it is essential that there be no retribution or negative consequences for staff.

Monitoring Staff Compensation Levels and Equity

"How Do I Ensure That Staff Compensation Is Equitable and Competitive?"

It is important for you to ensure that there is a periodic review of salaries and benefits for your departmental staff. If salaries are not competitive with those at other institutions, you can work with HR to correct the gaps. If inequities among staff are found, actions to correct these should be undertaken quickly [3]. Long-term employees may suffer from a "loyalty" tax and find that their compensation lags behind that of newer employees who were subsequently recruited at higher entry salaries [4]. Correction of these discrepancies is important for employee satisfaction, morale, and retention.

"What Are My Options if Compensation Is Below Market or Insufficient to Attract the Staff Talent I Need in My Department?"

A close working relationship with your institutional HR colleagues and other institutional leaders is useful to ensure competitive compensation for staff in your department. Ideally, these interactions will be proactively established rather than waiting for a problem to arise. Institutional data can be used to ensure that compensation and benefits for your departmental staff are comparable to those of staff in other parts of your AHC/AMC. Benchmarking data, both regional and national, also can identify compensation issues and be used to negotiate approvals of needed salary increases and augmented benefit packages.

Adjustments based on productivity and performance also are important considerations when considering total compensation [5]. It is often useful to calculate the direct and downstream expenses of raising compensation to competitive levels for longer retention of staff, in comparison to the ongoing recruitments needed to fill positions vacated due to below-market compensation. Beyond the impact to productivity, this financial comparison becomes very important when inadequate staffing leads to loss of revenue-generating activity (e.g., clinical services) or increased expenses (e.g., hourly contract employees).

"What Are the Challenges and Best Approaches to Having Both Staff (Nonfaculty) Physicians and Faculty Physicians in My Department?"

More AHCs/AMCs are hiring staff physicians who are not members of the salaried faculty due to the expansion of their health systems and with the goal of better meeting patient care needs (see also Chap. 17). These staff physicians may be employed by the hospital, faculty practice plan, or department. If staff physicians are members of your department, you should be cognizant of the differing roles and compensation between staff and faculty physicians, and articulate these to both constituencies. The use of metrics and reference to national standards for compensation can be useful. Articulating the need to maintain market competitiveness for staff physicians who could be providing identical services in private practice is important in considering how their salaries are set.

References

1. Society for Human Resource Management 2023. How to establish salary ranges. https://www. shrm.org/resourcesandtools/tools-and-samples/how-to-guides/pages/howtoestablishsala-ryranges.aspx. Accessed 29 Mar 2023.
2. Rodriguez JE, Campbell KM, Pololi LH. Addressing disparities in academic medicine: what of the minority tax? BMC Med Educ. 2015;15:1–5. https://doi.org/10.1186/s12909-015-0290-9.
3. Society for Human Resource Management 2023. Managing Pay Equity. https://www.shrm. org/resourcesandtools/tools-and-samples/toolkits/pages/managingpayequity.aspx. Accessed 29 Mar 2023.
4. Black E: You may be paying a "loyalty tax" at work. Here's why. Financ Rev. 2022. https:// www.afr.com/work-and-careers/workplace/you-may-be-paying-a-loyalty-tax-at-work-here-s-why-20221007-p5bnz8. Accessed 29 Mar 2023.
5. Society for Human Resource Management 2023. Performance and salary review policy. https://www.shrm.org/resourcesandtools/tools-and-samples/policies/pages/cms_000527.aspx. Accessed 29 Mar 2023.

Chapter 27
Dealing with Difficult or Unproductive Staff

Considerations

"When Should I Deal with Difficult or Unproductive Staff Personally and When Should I Involve Others?"

As chair, you should clearly establish which staff members directly report to you. This should be a small number of people, given the breadth of your supervisory and oversight responsibilities. In general, you should limit the number of staff for whom you act as immediate supervisor, which might include your chief administrator, your personal assistant, and perhaps a few key staff such as your head of finance and chief of staff. A clear-cut organizational chart for the remaining staff should be developed and practices put in place to ensure that reporting lines are understood by all staff and their supervisors.

For individuals reporting directly to you, you have primary responsibility for providing feedback on an ongoing basis. If performance difficulties arise, these should be discussed sooner rather than later and with full transparency. Be sure to lay out clear expectations for improvement, the manner in which they will be assessed, and advice on how to achieve success. If substantial, you may wish to involve an HR representative for advice, especially whether to have others present during difficult discussions. For staff who don't report directly to you, you should ensure that supervisors have the training needed to appropriately deal with challenging personnel issues.

In some cases, staff may approach you with complaints or concerns that they have not yet discussed with their supervisor. In general, it is best to encourage them to discuss their concerns with their supervisor first, but assure them that they have other options if they are not comfortable approaching their supervisor, including working with the HR department. You should not permit staff to leapfrog the system

F. Sanfilippo et al., *Lead, Inspire, Thrive*, https://doi.org/10.1007/978-3-031-41177-9_27

or attempt an end-around that avoids the prescribed approaches for resolution. Of course, you should ensure that the staff member is informed of the correct procedures and processes, including referral to appropriate resources in personnel manuals, websites, and the HR department. Consistency in communication and processes are important for equity, effective operations, and recognition of the appropriate role of supervisors.

Evaluation and Resolution

"What Policies Apply to Dealing with Staff Who Are Not Performing Well or Experiencing Personal or Interpersonal Issues?"

Your department should have equitable and transparent written standards for employee conduct and performance expectations that are aligned with institutional policies. This is critical to help employees understand the departmental culture and to achieve the greatest level of success possible in their jobs. It also provides the basis by which they can be evaluated.

When poor performance or disruptive behavior occurs, an assessment of the cause is an essential early step which should be made promptly. Questions to address include:

- Is the employee experiencing issues at home or with family members?
- Is there a physical or mental health reason for poor performance?
- Is the employee motivated to improve performance?
- Does the employee lack needed skill sets that could be addressed with additional training opportunities?

The answers to these questions should be fairly and objectively documented. Involvement of an expert from the institutional HR office or the school's ombudsperson may be helpful. Remember to consider whether the problem is that the job is a bad fit for the skills and interest of an otherwise good employee, and the best solution may be to change their jobs or responsibilities.

These and other insights can help guide how corrective policies are implemented and the specific actions taken. Outcomes that are fair to the employee, are fully compliant with policy and precedent, and benefit the department's operations are the goal. Remedial actions should be undertaken as soon as feasible with expectations clearly delineated.

"What Resources Are Available for Me to Help Staff Who Are Experiencing Difficulties in My Department?"

You should be sure that you, your leadership team, and staff supervisors know what internal and external resources are available to help staff improve performance. Institutional training programs can help increase staff members' confidence and engagement as well as teach them specific skills [1–4]. External training programs are available through professional organizations and can be used in a positive way to help employees achieve success and contribute effectively to the department. Provision of mentors or coaches can be helpful in some cases. Employee support services, ranging from mental health counseling to financial assistance, are available at many institutions and should be utilized as an important resource as needed by staff in your department.

"How Should Staff Performance Be Monitored in My Department?"

Periodic staff satisfaction surveys can provide important insights about your department, and exit interviews can reveal issues that need to be addressed [5]. Your HR department can assist with implementing and interpreting the results of these instruments. High employee turnover or low staff satisfaction scores usually indicate problems with departmental morale and culture. You should be aware of these results and share them with your leadership team and staff supervisors, maintaining appropriate attention to confidentiality.

Mistakes

"What Is the Best Approach to Deal with Staff Members Who Make Serious Mistakes in the Performance of Their Duties?"

Serious mistakes by staff members need to be compassionately and forthrightly addressed. As necessary, assistance should be requested from HR experts and others such as risk management officers and legal counsel depending on the nature of the mistake (e.g., clinical error, animal care violation). As chair, you need to ensure that issues are dealt with in a timely manner and that those with expertise in these matters have been appropriately involved. Careful documentation of all issues and interventions should be made and kept on file.

"How Do I Respond to Requests for Job References About Staff Who Have Left the Department Under Adverse Circumstances?"

Guidance from your HR department (and, if applicable, legal counsel) can help prevent you from missteps in these challenging situations. Disclosure of confidential information as well as incomplete disclosure can pose legal and ethical risks. If you unexpectedly receive a request for a reference (even from a friend or close colleague) about a staff member who has issues, consider getting advice from your institutional HR office or legal staff before responding.

References

1. Center for Creative Leadership: Why (and How) to Confront Difficult Employees. https://www.ccl.org/articles/leading-effectively-articles/confront-problem-employees/. Accessed 29 Mar 2023.
2. Gallo A. How to manage a toxic employee. Harv Bus Rev. 2016. https://hbr.org/2016/10/how-to-manage-a-toxic-employee. Accessed 29 Mar 2023.
3. McCormick J. The 8 types of difficult employees new managers struggle to lead. 2019. Leadership essentials. https://hcleadershipessentials.com/blogs/relationships-and-communication/8-types-of-difficult-employees-new-managers-struggle-to-lead. Accessed 29 Mar 2023.
4. Society for Human Resource Management: Managing Workplace Conflict. https://www.shrm.org/resourcesandtools/tools-and-samples/toolkits/pages/managingworkplaceconflict.aspx. Accessed 29 Mar 2023.
5. Webster J, Flint A. Exit interviews to reduce turnover amongst healthcare professionals. Cochrane Database Syst Rev. 2014;2014(8):CD006620. https://doi.org/10.1002/14651858.CD006620.pub4.

Part VII
Interactions Beyond Your Department

In addition to your activities in leading your department, your external interactions can have a significant impact on your success in meeting goals and expectations. Developing a good working relationship with institutional leaders is essential for you to be a team player on their leadership team, as is ensuring alignment of your departmental programs with institutional mission and priorities. Productive interactions with peer department and center leaders can facilitate the development of joint multidisciplinary programs of added value. Many opportunities for creating collaborative research, clinical, teaching, and public service programs exist beyond your institution, especially involving other universities, hospitals, professional societies, and nonprofit organizations that share your department's mission and values. Companies provide another set of opportunities for collaboration, usually through contractual arrangements that provide funding or other resources for research, clinical, or teaching services. Interactions with community leaders and the media also can provide significant benefits, especially by increasing visibility and recognition of people and programs.

Chapter 28
Interacting with Institutional Leaders

Understanding Your Institutional Leadership Teams

"What Should I Know About Leadership at My Institution(s)?"

It is important to understand your organization's leadership structure, relationships, and culture, which will help you determine with whom to interact for different issues and opportunities, as well as how to engage them effectively.

The first step in understanding the organization(s) with which you are directly involved (e.g., university, health system, private practice groups, clinics) is to understand their relationships and corporate models [e.g., not-for-profit versus for-profit, 501c3 public benefit corporation, limited liability company (LLC), partnership, others; see Chap. 2]. If you are involved with more than one institution, you also should determine their relationship to each other (e.g., ownership, partnership, affiliation, independent) and the nature of any operating or financial agreements among them. This information will provide you with insights about how they operate, their priorities, and how they are governed, all of which can impact your department directly or indirectly.

The next step is to understand the reporting relationships of your institutional leaders (e.g., dean, hospital director) and the teams that they lead. In some cases, deans have dual reports to the university president and provost for different activities and may also have a board to which they report. Hospital leaders usually report to a board but also may report to an independent AHC/AMC leader or university president. In some instances, one individual may hold several positions simultaneously (e.g., dean/AHC/AMC CEO; dean/health system chief academic officer; dean/university VP; health system CEO/AHC/AMC CEO). This information can provide insight on the level of authority these leaders have to make decisions independently (or together) that impact you and your department.

© The Author(s), under exclusive license to Springer Nature Switzerland AG 2023

F. Sanfilippo et al., *Lead, Inspire, Thrive*,

https://doi.org/10.1007/978-3-031-41177-9_28

A third step is to understand how these leaders' teams operate. Members of these teams are medical school and hospital senior staff, who may have significant delegated authority to make decisions that have implications for you and your department. Knowing when and how to interact with (or bypass) those you report to for appropriate issues can save time and effort for you, them, and their teams.

It is also important to understand the authority and responsibility of your peer department leaders as well as the leaders of other mission-based units (e.g., inter-, multidisciplinary centers, institutes, clinical services). Knowing when and how to engage your peer leaders to collaborate is critical for the resolution of issues involving shared resources and activities between your units and for creating new programs and initiatives.

A final (and to some extent the most important) understanding you should develop about your institutional leadership is their values and organizational culture (see Chap. 6). While it usually is easy to find the stated values of organizations in their strategic plans, it is much more difficult to determine their actual values in practice. In fact, when surveyed objectively, the culture and behavioral norms of AHCs/AMCs and their units often differ in actuality from what is stated [1, 2].

Working with Your Institutional Leaders

"How Do I Develop a Positive Relationship with Those to Whom I Report?"

Obviously, for the success of you personally as well as your department, it is critical to develop a positive relationship with all your supervisors and their teams. Since you likely were recruited and appointed by those to whom you report, your initial relationship with them should start out very positively. They have a vested interest in your success because they recruited you.

Important ways to develop a positive relationship with your supervisor(s) include [3]:

- Never try to go behind or around them to their superiors or board members without their knowledge, especially in a disagreement.
- Interact effectively and appropriately with their staff.
- Behave with them as you would want your own unit directors to behave with you.
- Be open and transparent.
- Do not meet only to make requests or resolve problems.
- Schedule regular meetings to share good news, departmental achievements, and your personal progress.
- Send or cc e-mails to them sparingly and carefully.
- Avoid giving them any surprises; provide a heads-up when a serious problem or significant benefit is looming.

In some cases, the recruitment of a department chair is handled by just one of two or more institutional leaders (e.g., a dean and hospital director), and there is little engagement and commitment by the other. In such cases, be sure to communicate with each of them and make it clear that your interests are to make each of their organizations successful.

When reporting to two or more bosses:

- Demonstrate engagement and commitment to the success of each of their institutions.
- Avoid taking sides when there is tension or disagreement among them.
- Be transparent with them if you are asked for a position on a contentious issue.
- Do not make requests that will benefit one at the expense of another.
- Promote alignment among all of the organizations to which you report.

"How Should I Bring Problems or Requests to My Bosses?"

It is important to understand the local culture and processes for resolving problems and requesting resources. Some useful tips for these interactions with your bosses include [3]:

- Don't bring them departmental conflicts for resolution; that is your job, not theirs.
- Be judicious and limit the number of problems or issues brought forward.
- Always provide a range of solutions to a problem and vet them beforehand with your leadership team and appropriate institutional leaders and staff.
- Be objective and dispassionate in a conflict and try to understand their points of view.
- Appreciate that they have many other priorities and limited resources.
- Always detail the benefits to the institution for a proposed departmental request or solution to a problem.
- Avoid bringing them surprises; if you anticipate an emerging problem or impending crisis, be sure to provide a heads-up to them or the appropriate members of their leadership teams.

Being a Team Player

"How Do I Balance My Role as Department Chair with Being an Institutional Team Player?"

As a department leader, remember that you also are considered to be part of the institutional leadership team. Department chairs effectively are middle managers and must represent the interests of both the institution and their department [4].

Strive to project your support of the whole institution, and that you are leading your department as an integral and supportive part of the institution(s). You and your department will benefit if you are viewed as a team player and a trusted colleague to your superiors.

The importance of teamwork cannot be overestimated [5]. Teamwork, accountability, and trust are key attributes in developing a constructive and collaborative relationship with your institutional leaders (bosses) and teammates (fellow chairs/directors). Position yourself and your department to be in win-win situations with your institution(s). Be a constructive critic and problem solver as appropriate, and try to improve the institution as well as your department.

References

1. Sanfilippo F, Bendapudi N, Rucci A, Schlesinger L. Strong leadership and teamwork drive culture and performance change: Ohio State University medical center 2000-2006. Acad Med. 2008;83:845–54. https://doi.org/10.1097/ACM.0b013e318181d2e7.
2. Sanfilippo F, Burns KH, Borowitz ML, Jackson JB, Hruban RH. The Johns Hopkins department of pathology novel organizational model: a 25-year ongoing experiment. Acad Pathol. 2018;5:2374289518811145. https://doi.org/10.1177/2374289518811145.
3. Sanfilippo F, Powell D, Folberg R, Tykocinski M. Dealing with deans and academic medical center leadership: advice from leaders. Acad Pathol. 2018;5:2374289518765462. https://doi.org/10.1177/2374289518765462.
4. Ness RB, Samet JM. How to be a department chair of epidemiology: a survival guide. Am J Epidemiol. 2010;172:747–51. https://doi.org/10.1093/aje/kwq268.
5. Kozlowski SWJ, Ilgen DR. Enhancing the effectiveness of work groups and teams. Psychol Sci Public Interest. 2006;7:77–124. https://doi.org/10.1111/j.1529-1006.2006.00030.x.

Chapter 29
Interdepartmental Interactions

Working with Peer Institutional Leaders

"How Can I Build Productive Relationships with My Peer Institutional Leaders?"

Personal relationships among peer leaders often take time to develop, can strongly influence departmental interactions, and are of many types. They can be mostly social, "one-offs," long-term strategic affiliations, or true partnerships built on shared values and trust. Relationships often progress from one type to another as they mature. If you have significant interactions with another department or program leader, consider extending your professional relationship with that leader to include a social one. Reciprocally, if you already have a personal-social relationship with another leader, consider how you might leverage your personal interactions to create collaborative programs and increased value for both of the units you are leading [1].

You should keep your peers as well as those to whom you report informed about the mission and accomplishments of your department. A useful way to promote interactions with another department/center/program is by scheduling joint conferences, seminars, and meetings to discuss areas of mutual interest. Institutional leadership meetings that include "update" presentations by departments can be very helpful in getting your message out and promoting your department's mission and vision, which can help expand departmental interactions and your relationship with other leaders. If your institution's leadership meetings don't include an opportunity for departments/centers/programs to share their activities, consider suggesting that it be added to the agenda as a regular item.

F. Sanfilippo et al., *Lead, Inspire, Thrive*,
https://doi.org/10.1007/978-3-031-41177-9_29

Developing Joint Programs

"What Are Ways to Build Synergistic Interdepartmental Programs?"

Interdepartmental programs can expand the scope and impact of your department's research, education, clinical, and outreach programs, as well as the efficiency and effectiveness of your administrative activities such as finance, HR, communications, and fundraising [2]. Your first step in developing any joint program is to identify areas of complementarity, duplication, or gaps between programs. Areas of complementarity provide the potential for creating joint programs with greater scope, while confronting duplication allows for potential efficiencies and scale. Addressing gaps between programs offers opportunities for developing new ones that can tie existing ones together.

Besides having greater impact, interdepartmental programs can improve communication, diminish competition among departments [3], and enhance fundraising opportunities (see Chap. 32). They can also result in recruitment of new talented faculty with shared academic appointments among participating departments/centers (see Chap. 17). The potential for developing synergistic interdepartmental programs spans all mission areas as well as administrative activities.

Clinical: Although interdepartmental clinical programs usually are developed and function as "product lines" in your health-care delivery system, you and other department/center leaders can often identify ways to enhance these programs by soliciting suggestions from your faculty and staff and evaluating departmental revenues and expenses. Recommendations to institutional leaders about developing or changing interdepartmental clinical programs should always be a joint effort among the department leaders involved, with a bottom line of how such changes will impact patients, faculty, trainees, and staff, as well as the anticipated financial impact on the institution and the departments involved. How resources are contributed and benefits distributed among all parties should be equitable and transparent (see below and Chap. 10).

Research: The impact and importance of interdisciplinary research is enormous and has become a major source of innovation. Most AHCs/AMCs have centers and institutes that leverage research disciplines with clinical specialties, most notably in cancer and cardiovascular disease, as well as more basic multidisciplinary research programs in areas such as molecular genetics, biomedical engineering, and data science-bioinformatics.

There likely are many opportunities to expand your department's research activities with others at the level of individual faculty collaborations. Faculty involved in basic, clinical, translational, and health services research in your department can often add value to many of these areas in other departments. Identifying and promoting interdisciplinary and interdepartmental opportunities to your faculty will help make it happen. Likewise, leveraging multi-investigator research programs in your department with those in others through your leadership relationships can become the basis for creating new institutional programs, centers, and institutes that will provide access to resources not otherwise available.

Education: Many professional health education programs have become more multi-departmental (and even multi-institutional) over the past decade and have engaged disciplines previously outside the health sciences (e.g., data science, engineering, business, social sciences). Multi-degree offerings (e.g., MD-PhD, MD-MBA, MD-MPH, MD-JD), training programs, fellowships, and continuing education programs have greatly expanded the disciplines involved and the interests of learners. Among other benefits, you can expand your department's reach to a broader range of scholars by being involved in the development and delivery of these programs.

As discussed previously, the most effective way to build interdepartmental programs in education, as well as health-care delivery, research, and public service is by stimulating collaboration (see Chap. 8, section "Stimulating Collaboration") and providing appropriate incentives (see Chap. 19, section "Incentives and Bonuses").

Public service: The public service mission of most medical school departments includes participation and support of local and regional community benefit activities, which can be enhanced by interdisciplinary/interdepartmental programs and involve faculty, staff, and student participation. Examples are most common in working with public and community health services to help provide comprehensive diagnostic and clinical services to the underserved and with local schools to help provide health education lectures and courses. Of course, there are many other areas of public service that can engage your department to increase the benefits provided; the key is a willingness to collaborate if approached and proactively look for partnership opportunities.

Administrative: In addition to interdepartmental programs driven by missions, you should consider how to improve administrative productivity in your department by developing shared resources with other departments. If your department is small and unable to adequately support your desired needs in key areas (e.g., finance, IT, HR, communications), it can be mutually beneficial to develop cross-departmental programs. Reciprocally, if you have excess administrative capacity in some areas, it is worth finding departments that can use it. Developing or expanding shared services (e.g., diagnostic labs, research core facilities, teaching technologies) with other departments/centers can also be of substantial value (see Chap. 13, section "People"). Financial benefits, greater technical expertise, and increased productivity are among the important measures to document as you build successful shared-service programs.

Remember that in many cases excellent opportunities to collaborate exist with departments and centers beyond your medical school in your AHC/AMC and university, as well as with other organizations (see Chap. 31) which often can provide unique resources that can enrich and complement your own department's programs.

Resources and Recognition

"How Can I Best Obtain and Use Resources for Interdepartmental Programs?"

As discussed above and in Chap. 13, the key to obtaining resources for joint programs is by demonstrating the benefits to all stakeholders, including participating departments, the institution, and those being served. Moreover, the distribution of benefits should be equitable and transparent (see Chap. 10).

Often the most difficult part of developing interdepartmental programs is how to trade off different types of resource contributions (e.g., space by one department, personnel and funding by others). Likewise, the benefits may vary among participants (e.g., greater clinical activity/revenue in one department, research activity/ grants in another). Trying to agree on an exactly equal distribution of resources and benefits can often kill the creation of joint programs and hurt personal relationships among parties. Remember that perfect is often the enemy of good!

In considering resources, you should simply try to ensure that all parties have some net benefit return on what they contribute (including good will and future consideration), and not be completely focused on how much each party gets. Your reputation with peers and superiors, and success as a leader, can be enhanced by being recognized as someone who is always interested in creating more value for all rather than trying to get the most benefit for yourself. This approach will open more opportunities for developing joint departmental programs and greater success for you and your department.

Similarly, recognition of contributions made by you and your department in developing joint programs is important, but it's even more important to get the programs implemented, which may mean staying in the background if recognition is more important to other participants. To paraphrase what has been said by many great leaders (including Harry Truman and Ronald Reagan): "You can accomplish almost anything if you don't worry about who gets the credit."

"How Can I Best Promote the 'Purview' of My Department in a Constructive Manner and Without Offending Colleagues in Other Departments?"

You should clearly articulate your department's mission, activities, and achievements so that your peer leaders understand and appreciate your department. However, the rapid increase in knowledge and technology, especially over the past decade, has substantially expanded the education, clinical, research, and outreach activities for most health science disciplines, resulting in substantially more overlap among departments within and outside AHCs/AMCs. Moreover, this has led to the creation of new departments that have assumed activities previously in other departments. As a result, there are essentially no basic science or clinical departments that don't overlap in their activities and interests with other departments. The beneficial effect of this trend has been the creation of many more interdisciplinary centers and institutes, as well as greater opportunities for joint interdepartmental programs (see above).

Unfortunately, in some cases the overlap in the activities of departments and centers results in competition and conflict for patients, students, faculty, resources, and recognition. When promoting the activities of your department, it is important to be sensitive to areas of overlap and actual competition with other departments by not being negative or comparative about their programs. As appropriate, it is highly constructive to positively mention overlapping and competing programs as an alternative option to what your department offers, especially to potential patients and students. Ideally, this will be reciprocated and provide greater benefit to all.

Dealing with Interdepartmental Conflicts

"How Should I Deal with Conflicts Between My Department and Other Departments and Centers?"

Conflicts among departments/centers/units are among the most challenging issues facing leaders and often involve financial, programmatic, personnel, or operational issues. They may vary according to the source of the conflict (faculty, staff, leader) and the magnitude of the impact on the departments involved and parent institution(s). Conflicts among peer units can affect their success [4] and if unresolved can expand to broader discord affecting other relationships and the parent institution(s).

In dealing with intra-institutional conflicts, you should understand the nature of the conflict in detail and the vested interests of those involved [5]. Attempts at negotiating a resolution should be informal at first, involving you and the peer leader of the conflicting unit (see Chap. 10). If informal resolution is not possible, the nature and details of the conflict should be documented in writing and, as needed, escalated to the institutional officials responsible for the pertinent areas. For serious conflicts, some institutions may use professional conflict-resolution experts. The influence of a strong institutional leader is often necessary to mitigate conflict, and conflicts may be prolonged or remain unresolved with weak (e.g., interim) or disinterested (e.g., overwhelmed) institutional leaders. In all cases, you should try to prevent departmental conflicts from harming your personal relationships with your peers and institutional leaders.

References

1. Pogue S. 11 ways to improve collaboration between departments. 2022. https://www.workzone.com/blog/9-ways-to-improve-collaboration-between-departments/. Accessed 29 Mar 2023.
2. Mallon WT, Grigsby RK. Leading: top skills, attributes, and behaviors critical for success. Washington, DC: Association of American Medical Colleges; 2016. ISBN 978-1577541509.
3. Willett CG. Reflections from a chair: leadership of a clinical department at an academic medical center. Cancer. 2015;22:3795–8. https://doi.org/10.1002/cncr.29588.
4. Menon A, Jaworski BJ, Kohli AK. Product quality: impact of interdepartmental interactions. J Acad Mark Sci. 1997;25:187–200. https://doi.org/10.1177/0092070397253001.
5. American Management Association: The five steps to conflict resolution. 2023. https://www.amanet.org/articles/the-five-steps-to-conflict-resolution/. Accessed 29 Mar 2023.

Chapter 30
Departmental and Institutional Alignment

Determining Priorities

"How Should I Determine the Appropriate Priorities for My Department?"

As an institutional leader you need to know your institution and should fully understand and embrace its mission, values, and vision [1]. As a department chair you should be sure that they are well understood by your faculty and staff and are consistent (but not necessarily duplicative) with the priorities and expectations of your department (see Chap. 3). A good understanding of institutional and departmental mission, vision, values, and expectations by you and your faculty and staff will help assure that the priorities and goals developed by your strategic planning process are appropriate (see Chap. 12).

Although the mission, vision, values, and expectations of two independent parent institutions (e.g., school/university and hospital/health system) usually differ (e.g., scholarship versus patient care), they can be coordinated and in alignment as an AHC/AMC, especially in clinical education and training as well as clinical and health services research. However, it is difficult to align your departmental priorities with parent institutions that are not aligned with each other. In these situations, you must try to develop a bimodal approach in setting goals and priorities to satisfy the expectations of the two (or more) entities.

F. Sanfilippo et al., *Lead, Inspire, Thrive*,
https://doi.org/10.1007/978-3-031-41177-9_30

Misalignment with Institutional Mission and Vision

"How Should I Deal with Misalignment of My Department Mission and Vision with Those of a Parent Institution?"

If the mission and vision of your department are incompatible with those of a parent institution, conflict likely will follow because of the inevitable inconsistency in strategic priorities, goals, and expectations. These disparities may persist in situations where your institution(s) have extensive resources, redundant departments and disciplines, or more pressing priorities. However, in most cases, you ultimately will lose support in both resources and your relationships with leaders if the strategic priorities and goals of your department are not aligned with the mission and expectations of your institution(s).

If recognized as a problem by your institutional leadership, and not resolved in a timely manner, misalignment will often result in micromanagement of your department and potentially your dismissal as chair. Therefore, if you begin to feel that your departmental mission and priorities are not aligning with those of your institution(s), you should quickly seek the advice and help of institutional leaders and other advisors (especially from outside the department who will be more objective) to determine the causes and how to resolve the misalignment (see Chap. 34).

Building Alignment

"How Can I Build Alignment Between My Department and Institutional Leadership Regarding Mission and Vision?"

Assuring alignment between your department and parent institution(s) begins at the start of your strategic planning process in defining mission, values, and vision as the context for determining your department's goals and priorities (see Chap. 12). In cases where departmental and institutional alignment is ambiguous, outside consultants are often helpful. When conflict exists between parent institutions (e.g., school/university and hospital/health system), it is difficult to align departmental mission, vision, and values with two (or more) entities that are not themselves aligned. As mentioned above for priorities, in these situations you must develop a dual approach of alignment with both institutions.

Over the past decade, most AHCs/AMCs have tried to align their clinical, research, education, and public service missions, even when split between different institutions. In some cases, this has been facilitated by structural changes at the institutional leadership level by combining functions and positions under a single leader to oversee the entire AHC/AMC leadership team [2]. The past decade has also seen increased alignment of clinical service activities under the health systems,

so that in many cases, clinical practice plans that had been in the medical school/
university have moved into the hospital/health system, even when involving separate corporate entities.

Even more effective than structural integration is functional alignment of medical schools and teaching hospitals through their leadership behavior, relationships, and decision-making [3, 4]. These organizational alignments can improve communication, which is the basis for achieving understanding, trust, and collaboration (see Chaps. 5 and 8).

"How Should I Deal with Changes in Institutional Priorities and Use of Resources?"

It is important for you to appreciate, and help your department understand, that AHCs/AMCs usually consider department resources, especially funds and space, as their own. Since your department is only part of the enterprise, your institution(s) may have better opportunities and higher priorities for use of those resources. Difficult as it may be to achieve, this understanding will help build alignment [5]. However, by embracing this philosophy, you may (at least initially) be viewed by your departmental faculty and staff as giving in to ingratiate yourself to institutional leaders.

It takes courage to stand with the institution when on the surface or in the short term it may not seem to be in the best interest of the department. It is incumbent upon you to explain to your department faculty and staff that in most cases "what is good for the institution is ultimately good for the department." It may be helpful to involve institutional leadership in discussions with your faculty and staff about how benefiting the institution overall ultimately should help the department and its members. Communicating effectively with institutional leaders and your department is the key to rebuilding alignment when there are changes in institutional priorities (see Chap. 5, section "Accommodating Institutional Priorities and Reforms").

References

1. Fisher M. Being chair: a 12-step program for medical school chairs. Int J Med Educ. 2011;2:147–51. https://doi.org/10.5116/ijme.4ece.862d.
2. Sanfilippo F, Bendapudi N, Rucci A, Schlesinger L. Strong leadership and teamwork drive culture and performance change: Ohio State University medical center 2000-2006. Acad Med. 2008;83:845–54. https://doi.org/10.1097/ACM.0b013e318181d2e7.
3. Keroack MS, McConkie NR, Johnson EK, Epting J, Thompson IM, Sanfilippo F. Functional alignment, not structural integration, of medical schools and their teaching hospitals is associated with performance in academic health centers. Am J Surg. 2011;202:119–26. https://doi.org/10.1016/j.amjsurg.2011.05.001.

4. Rouse WB, Cortese DA. Engineering the system of healthcare delivery. In: Health system: information knowledge systems management. Amsterdam: IOS Press; 2010. ISBN 978-1607505310.
5. Bailey DN, Crawford JM, Jensen PE, Leonard DGB, McCarthy S, Sanfilippo F. Generating discretionary income in an academic department of pathology. Acad Pathol. 2021;8:23742895211044811. https://doi.org/10.1177/23742895211044811.

Chapter 31
Interactions with External Entities

Getting Institutional Approval

"When and How Should I Get Institutional Approval for External Interactions?"

The first step before considering interactions with external entities is to understand the general policies and practices of your institution(s) regarding communication with other organizations, especially concerning conflicts of interest, nondisclosure agreements, and preexisting relationships. In addition, it is useful to understand the approval process for any agreement that might result from an interaction, and determine beforehand if it is worth the potential time and effort needed to execute a program.

In most cases the policies, practices, and agreement processes will differ for the different types of entities discussed below, based on whether they are a potential/actual competitor, a for-profit or not-for-profit entity, or an individual rather than an organization. You likely will need to engage with your institutional legal, communications/marketing, and risk management offices in developing and implementing external agreements, which can become very complicated if you have two or more parent institutions.

© The Author(s), under exclusive license to Springer Nature
Switzerland AG 2023
F. Sanfilippo et al., *Lead, Inspire, Thrive*,
https://doi.org/10.1007/978-3-031-41177-9_31

Universities

"How Can I Take Advantage of Potential Opportunities for My Department with Other Universities?"

Many department chairs develop relationships with other universities through collaboration with peer leaders to develop joint programs. This is especially true when a local/regional university has health sciences (e.g., nursing, pharmacy, public health, veterinary medicine) or other academic programs (e.g., business, engineering, social work) that are not at your parent institution(s). Such potential collaborative relationships predominantly are in research (e.g., multicenter grants, shared core lab services) and education (e.g., multidisciplinary training programs, combined degrees, joint CME courses).

The key to creating inter-institutional collaborative programs is developing a trusting relationship with leaders at the partner university who share values and priorities (see Chap. 8). The best way for you to make this happen is by spending time with them on their turf and inviting them to spend time on yours. Allowing appropriate adjunct appointments for faculty at both institutions can strengthen these relationships and help identify other potential opportunities (see Chap. 17). Another essential part of building and sustaining trust is negotiating mutually beneficial terms for the programs developed and their participants (see Chap. 10).

"What Issues Should I Consider When Interacting with Other Universities?"

Obviously, developing joint programs with other institutions should provide your department with some net benefits when considering the actual and opportunity costs. Unfortunately, partnerships with other university programs can sometimes become problematic, especially when institutional conditions or leaders change. One example is when negotiated terms become disproportionally unsatisfactory to you because of unanticipated factors, and there is resistance to change the agreement. Another is when a new leader of the partner program has less interest in its success. The change may even be on your side, for example, when you have the opportunity to develop other programs of higher priority that would use fewer resources to sustain.

Regardless of the cause, if joint programs stop providing expected value, you should be candid and collegial in approaching their leaders to discuss the situation. All perspectives should be taken into consideration, as well as all options, including renegotiation, suspension, or termination of the program. Be sure your discussion concludes on a positive note, as it will reflect on your reputation and leave open the possibility of future agreements.

Hospitals and Health Systems

"What Are the Major Considerations When Interacting with Hospitals?"

AHCs/AMCs have many different models of interactions between medical schools and hospitals (see Chap. 2). In many cases, medical schools (or their parent university) own the hospital, while in other instances, medical schools have affiliations with one or more hospitals, clinics, or other patient care entities. When the medical school and hospital have common governance, department chairs usually have a defined role in the hospital (e.g., service chief, etc.) and thus may have dual reporting to the dean and to the hospital CEO. When an affiliated hospital is independent of a university-based medical school, the medical school department chair usually has to interact and negotiate with the affiliated hospital's leadership and may or may not have a formal hospital title and explicit responsibilities. As chair, it is essential that you understand the model at your AHC/AMC, the lines of governance and authority, and the implications for you and your faculty, staff, trainees, and students.

"How Can I Take Advantage of Potential Opportunities at Other Hospitals?"

There often are opportunities to develop collaborative programs at hospitals beyond those with which you have a primary affiliation. These usually involve local or regional community hospitals or clinics, which may be sites for medical student and resident education, participation in clinical trials and health services research, and providing clinical consultation support. Independent specialty hospitals (e.g., pediatrics, cancer, orthopedics) are important potential partners as they often have clinical, education, and research opportunities that are not available at your AHC/AMC and vice versa. As with developing joint university programs (see above), the key to working with other hospitals/clinics is to have trusted partners and equitable agreements with a clear understanding of potential conflicts, especially if the other hospital is in competition with your primary affiliated hospital for patients, recognition (i.e., marketing), or revenue.

"What Are Some of the Risks of Interacting with Other Hospitals?"

One of the major risks with programs at hospitals or clinics other than your primary affiliate(s) is if your faculty or staff members become a recruitment target by the other institution to build their own independent program. This is not uncommon, and you should carefully consider including noncompete clauses in your agreements as a way to help mitigate such poaching, with the understanding that these clauses cannot completely prevent it. The reciprocal also occurs, whereby faculty/staff from the partner hospital become your targets for recruitment; in either case, such activities usually will destroy the program partnership and have serious repercussions throughout both institutions and the broader community.

Another significant risk with joint programs at another hospital is to the brand of your department and your parent institution(s). Occasionally a community hospital with a joint program will market itself as having the same attributes as an AMC, but with easier access and lower costs. This can become even more problematic when the local hospital also has an affiliation with a national "name-brand" institution that they also market. You should be sure that your program agreement clearly spells out how the use of names and brands is allowed. You also should include exit clauses in your agreements that can be executed quickly to deal with some of these problems, which can occur suddenly without warning.

"Are There Special Hospital Affiliations That I Should Consider for My Department?"

For many medical schools, the Veterans Health Affairs Health Care System provides major sources of educational material for students and trainees as well as a supportive environment for clinical and research faculty in many disciplines. In fact, affiliations between these two institutions have been spelled out as a federal policy objective since 1946 [1]. Similarly, affiliations between medical schools and children's hospitals have enriched training for medical students, residents, and fellows, as well as research and clinical opportunities for faculty, even in those medical schools in which there is a pediatric service [2]. Another more specific example is for communities and states with independent medical examiner's offices, which require an affiliation to provide training to meet forensic pathology board certification requirements [3].

Professional Societies

"How Can I Take Advantage of Working with Professional Societies?"

Since you and most of your department's faculty and senior staff are members of associations and societies in your professions, these relationships can be used to identify, develop, and participate in mutually beneficial projects and programs.

Activities with professional societies also can provide substantial recognition for involved faculty and staff to help their career advancement. For faculty, these most often involve societies focused on the clinical, research, and education in their areas of specialty, as well as major national organizations that span all biomedical disciplines including the AAMC, AHA (American Hospital Association), and AMA. Many professional organizations have substantial resources to sponsor and support research, education, and clinical and public service-oriented projects that you and your faculty might develop.

For staff, numerous societies and organizations exist in virtually every area of operations and administration. Although most of these are business-oriented and dominated by membership from outside academic medicine, there are some specialty societies specifically for AHC/AMC administrative staff, such as in IT, development/fundraising, and communications. These are particularly useful in helping staff access resources and colleagues who can assist in identifying appropriate benchmarks and developing best practices.

"What Are Some of the Issues to Consider with Professional Society Interactions?"

Although involvement of you and your faculty and staff with professional organizations can provide substantial benefits and recognition, these relationships may be at the expense of your department. The time and effort for faculty and staff volunteer work with their professional organizations is usually not counted against consulting or vacation time, so it is effectively subsidized by the department. Moreover, some activities, especially development of educational tools and products, may generate revenue that goes to the professional organization even though the faculty/staff time (and often the resources for creating these products) is at the expense of the department.

Significant conflict of interest and commitment problems can arise if your faculty or staff have agreements or contracts for activities that are outside of your department without appropriate approvals, especially if they involve intellectual property. This will also become your problem with institutional leaders for not knowing about the situation and not ensuring that processes were in place to prevent it. You should be sure that you and your faculty and staff are well aware of how to interact with their professional organizations, and how conflict of interest and commitment as well as intellectual property policies may apply to you and them (see Chap. 33, section "Handling Conflicts of Interest").

As department chair you may feel obligated to attend as many professional society meetings as possible in order to maintain the visibility of your department, considering it to be your "professional duty." However, you must weigh the advantages of such visibility against the disadvantages (real or perceived) of having an apparent conflict of commitment by being an "absentee," "travelling," or "out-of-touch" chair who does not have a hand on the pulse of the department. Be sure that the occasional definition of "full-time" faculty as meaning traveling full time is not associated with you!

Non-Profit Organizations

"What Are Issues to Consider in Working with Non-Profit Organizations?"

Non-profit organizations include a wide range of entities that exist for the public benefit including professional and specialty societies (see above), non-governmental organization (NGOs), and philanthropic foundations. Almost all AHCs/AMCs include universities, medical and other professional schools, hospitals, and clinics that are non-profit organizations with a shared interest in the public benefit and are thus motivated to create many opportunities for partnerships of mutual benefit. A wide range of non-profit organizations and NGOs also provide funding support for projects that may be of interest, especially in developing policy through health services research [4].

Unfortunately, a common problem with projects from non-profit organizations is that the grants (and cost recovery) supporting them have a much lower indirect cost rate than for government grants. Before accepting grants from non-profits, you should be sure to consider the full financial impact of these projects on your department and institution. The unanticipated expense in time and money may make them less attractive than initially apparent.

Companies

"How Can My Department Take Advantage of Working with For-Profit Companies?"

Traditionally, corporate interactions have provided significant benefits to AHCs/AMCs by engaging them at the cutting edge of biomedical technology research and development of diagnostic and therapeutic devices and product, as well as the creation of educational products, and sponsorship of clinical trials. More recently, the rapid evolution of consumer-oriented services using virtual technology in clinical care (e.g., Sharecare, Amwell) and education (e.g., Coursera, Udacity) has created even more opportunities to work with companies. In many cases companies will seek out faculty and programs to work on specific programs.

Although there are many similarities in developing programs with companies and non-profit organizations, there are significant differences. Unlike relationships with non-profits, which can be true partnerships with shared values, corporations must prioritize financial profit and shareholder value, resulting in interactions that normally represent a vendor-client relationship. Likewise, there usually are differences in how program agreements are executed with corporations compared with non-profit organizations. All corporate agreements require a legal review of terms, especially to identify conflicts of interest, resources provided, payments and commitments of both parties, ownership of intellectual property, and allocation of revenue.

A major consideration of companies in developing relationships with AHC/AMC faculty and programs is the ease of working with the institution to finalize these agreements. Overly bureaucratic processes at some institutions significantly dampen corporate interest. You can help develop corporate opportunities for your department by facilitating the agreement process at your institution (e.g., help develop standardized approval processes, creation of templated master agreements) and especially by demonstrating prior examples of successful corporate interactions.

"What Are Some of the Risks and Problems of Working with Companies?"

Working with companies provides many of the same issues as discussed above with professional societies and non-profit organizations. These issues need to be carefully addressed before finalizing an agreement, especially those involving potential conflicts of interest, use and distribution of resources and benefits, and use of brand. In particular, the involvement of your faculty in clinical and educational services programs can create significant problems in all these areas if not properly identified and managed. You (or your designee) should be aware of the online rosters of corporate service vendors to make sure the involvement of any of your faculty is appropriate.

Community Leaders

"How Can I Best Engage Productively with Community Leaders?"

Community leaders represent all sectors of a region and can be a major source of support for your parent institution(s), especially as philanthropic donors and members of university and hospital governance and advisory boards. As board members involved in approving institutional priorities and resource allocations, their recognition of your department's activities, achievements, and value to the institution is very important. Moreover, having a positive personal relationship with board members will reflect well on your department and the institutional leaders who recruited you.

Developing positive relationships with community leaders, whether in a governance role or not, also can be of direct value to you and your department. Their business and other professional activities may provide opportunities to identify or facilitate interactions with external organizations as discussed above. They also can be very helpful in the recruitment of high-profile candidates for positions in clinical, education, or research areas in which they have a personal interest. Moreover, they often will help fund such programs through their own philanthropy or by helping to raise funds from others. The experiences of successful leaders in your community also can be very helpful in providing personal advice for your own leadership decisions (see Chap. 34).

The key to developing relationships with community leaders is the same as with anyone else; you have to spend time to get to know them, and for them to know you. For those involved in your institution, make sure to attend meetings and functions where they are present. However, probably the best way to develop these relationships is by attending the community functions that they attend and supporting areas of their community interest outside the AHC/AMC.

"What Are Some of the Risks and Problems in Dealing with Community Leaders?"

As discussed previously (see Chaps. 20 and 27), a major problem is when a faculty/ staff member with a close relationship to a community leader uses it to try to influence your oversight of their activities. This can become very difficult, especially if the community leader has a relationship with institutional leader(s) and engages directly with them on behalf of a problem faculty/staff member. In some cases, pushing back on the faculty/staff member for this behavior will only exacerbate the problem, as they will press the community member to become even more involved.

If the community leader has raised the issue of a faculty/staff member with those to whom you report, your first step is to discuss the situation with them for advice and assistance. Ideally, the institutional leader(s) will respond appropriately to the community leader and may arrange a meeting for you both with the community member to help explain and resolve the situation. If the community leader only has raised the issue with you, it is still wise to inform your institutional leaders before reacting to avoid any surprises and get their advice and, if appropriate, their assistance.

If the pressure by a community leader on your institutional leaders results in their support of the "end-around" by a faculty/staff member in your department who clearly has violated a procedure, process, behavioral standard, or agreement, it is time for you to consider a transition to another position (see Chap. 37, section

"Knowing When It's Time"). Naturally, you should never use your relationship with community leaders to "end-around" your own institutional leader(s); the repercussions likely would result in another good reason for you to consider transitioning!

The Media

"How Do I Best Engage with the Media?"

Dealing with the media in many ways is similar to dealing with community leaders, but on a magnified scale. Since only a portion of community leaders control the media and influence their content and editorial slant, your relationships with leaders and the media can be synergistic but sometimes antagonistic. Clearly the media has great impact in providing broad recognition to the local or national community about programs, activities, and individuals at your institution(s), which can be very beneficial or detrimental [5].

Most medical schools and parent institutions have significant marketing and advertising activities with the local (and sometimes national) media, as well as extensive interactions through institutional offices of communication and community affairs. The best way for you to interact with the media is through these offices. If you or your department has an item you believe to be newsworthy, share it first with your institutional media experts for their advice on if and how to bring it forward. Often it is best to have the story developed by your institutional media and sent as a press release to the external media.

In some cases, you may be contacted directly by the media regarding an achievement or activity by you or an individual or program in your department that they feel could be newsworthy. While it is tempting to work with them directly, it is better to involve your institutional experts to provide an interface that could be useful if the resulting story is inaccurate or negative. Likewise, you may be contacted by the media to be interviewed for an opinion or to comment on a news item they are working on. Although flattering and tempting, it again is wise to delay a response long enough to engage your institutional media experts who can better anticipate potential risks and benefits of providing an opinion or commentary on a specific issue.

"What Are Some of the Risks and Problems in Dealing with the Media?"

As with any company, you should always remember that the bottom line for the media is to generate profits, which is done by successfully competing with other media by selling more advertising, subscriptions, and, increasingly important in the

Internet world, getting more "clicks." Unfortunately, this has created much more "fake news" as a profit-making vehicle for some media outlets and resulted in a greater focus on being sensational rather than just factual and being politicized rather than neutral. The result has been that the risks of your comments being misrepresented and taken out of context have increased substantially, and factors such as the public perception of the political slant of the particular media outlet can negatively impact your reputation. Also, as most leaders learn eventually, what is actually released by the media from an interview may often differ significantly from what was expected.

Unfortunately, some media organizations (usually out of the mainstream) are entirely focused on reporting gossip and innuendo and routinely misrepresent issues by omission or commission. Their tactics may include Freedom of Information Act (FOIA) requests for records such as e-mails, which can be distressing and time-consuming if you are at an institution that must comply. Personal attacks on visible leaders by such media are generally recognized at face value by most people in the community, but nonetheless can be very hurtful if you are the target (see Chap. 33, section "Dealing with Criticism"). While they beg for an appropriate response, it is usually best for you to ignore such stories, since responding to them gives them more credibility and stimulates more stories and public interest. As is often said, no one comes out of a mud fight feeling clean, so just walking away is usually the best response. However, it again is important to get the advice of your communications and public relations (PR) experts before deciding on how to react.

References

1. Bailey DN. Academic pathology departments and associated children's hospitals: an overview of the relationship. Acad Pathol. 2020a;7:2374289520964935. https://doi.org/10.1177/2374289520964935.
2. Bailey DN. The veterans affairs healthcare system and academic pathology departments: evaluation of the relationship. Acad Pathol. 2020;7:2374289520939265. https://doi.org/10.1177/2374289520939265.
3. Bailey DN. The relationship between medical-school based pathology departments and affiliated forensic pathology training sites. Acad Pathol. 2021;8:23742895211040208. https://doi.org/10.1177/23742895211040208.
4. Pomeroy C, Sanfilippo F. How research can and should inform public policy. In: Wartman SA, editor. The transformation of academic health centers: meeting the challenges of healthcare's changing landscape. London: Elsevier; 2015. p. 179–91. ISBN 978-0128007624.
5. Larsson A, Appel S, Sundberg CJ, Rosenqvist M. Medicine and the media: medical experts' problems and solutions while working with journalists. PLoS One. 2019;14:e0220897. https://doi.org/10.1371/journal.pone.0220897.

Chapter 32
Fundraising and Donor Development

Identifying Uses

"What Activities Should I Target for Departmental Fundraising?"

Gifts provided as discretionary (unrestricted) funds are clearly the most flexible and desirable [1]. However, in most cases, potential donors and foundations will identify specific activities they wish to support. Obviously, it is best to target departmental fundraising for the programs identified as priorities in your strategic plan, especially for those that are under-resourced.

Donors often wish to establish endowments to support ongoing activities in areas of their interest that are led by individuals they know and respect. These endowments can include support for faculty chairs, student scholarships/fellowships, research programs, awards, lectureships, specific departmental programs/initiatives, and discretionary use. Frequently, donors want to name the endowed entity in recognition of their family or an important figure in their life. While the department should allow maximum flexibility in these naming opportunities, you must be careful about allowing names that may be controversial and may not reflect well upon the institution, the school, and the department.

In contrast to funding endowments, some donors prefer having their contributions be fully expended on an activity over a limited time to see more impact sooner. This approach often includes one-time funding for space or equipment that supports clinical service, research, or teaching activities.

Donors also often want to provide gifts that leverage existing resources. Particularly attractive are donor-matching programs. They also like to provide gifts that really "make a difference," enabling a high impact program to develop that otherwise would not.

F. Sanfilippo et al., *Lead, Inspire, Thrive*, https://doi.org/10.1007/978-3-031-41177-9_32

"What Activities Should I Avoid for Departmental Fundraising?"

Although gifts may appear similar in dollar amount, you should avoid the ones that create additional ongoing expenses for the department (i.e., "gifts that keep on costing"). This can happen when a gift requires, but does not fund, substantial personnel effort (especially faculty/senior staff), operating costs, or facility and equipment maintenance expenses. Such gifts may end up costing the department much more than the gift itself, especially over time.

Gifts that fully fund nonpriority activities may not seem to add additional expenses, but you should consider the time and opportunity costs involved when evaluating such potential donations. You also should avoid soliciting donations for operating or administrative expenses, since most donors rightfully consider these to be an institutional responsibility and not a good use of their contributions.

The department must remain true to its core mission and values; accordingly, you should not accept gifts that run counter to its mission and values. Similarly, you should not accept gifts to launch programs that are not aligned with your departmental strategic plan unless they are of a magnitude to fully support all the resource needs for development and sustained maintenance of the program.

Gifts to establish endowed professorships/chairs/scholarships must not be accepted when the donor believes they have the ability to select recipients. Their input should be welcomed but institutional policies must govern the actual selection process. Although grateful patients often wish to honor their physician (sometimes after encouragement by that physician), the institution's established process for such selection also must be followed. This will mitigate against grateful patients feeling that they have "purchased" a physician who must be available to them at all times.

Developing Donors

"How Should I Engage Potential Donors?"

The key to fundraising is developing strong relationships with potential donors to determine their areas of interest and educating them about the activities of the department that might align with those interests. In addition, sharing professional and social interests can go a long way in building strong relationships with potential donors. Most sophisticated donors consider their contributions to be investments and therefore will evaluate the commitment and competency of the leader involved in the program they fund, and also will want to understand the potential impact of the program to assess the return on their gift. Since most donations are dependent on a trusting relationship with the department or program leader, always think to "develop the relationship first, discuss the donation second."

Educating potential donors about the activities, successes, ambitions, and potential impact of the department and identifying specific areas of their interest is a process that often takes years to develop, which is why fundraising is called "development." Moreover, many donors think that research, clinical service, and teaching each generate profit margins, so it often is useful to educate them about the amount of unrecovered research costs, the extent of low and uncompensated clinical services, and the student tuition burden at your AHC/AMC.

For departments with little or no direct patient contact, it may be helpful for the department chair to partner with leaders of patient-facing departments/centers in development efforts, especially if together they can create interdisciplinary programs that benefit all involved (see Chap. 29, section "Developing Joint Programs"). Some common examples of interdisciplinary programs among departments/centers that attract donors include cancer, heart disease, children's health, infectious diseases, informatics, and genetics.

It may be helpful to establish a department "Board of Visitors (or Advisors)" consisting of past and potential donors as a way of enhancing the visibility of you and your department. It is well recognized that your best potential donors are your past donors, and mixing past donors with potential ones can help stimulate more contributions from all of them. You can engage the group through social events, communication, and regularly scheduled meetings to discuss and solicit their informal feedback and advice on the activities, needs, and opportunities in the department. However, you should be careful that such a board does not consider itself to have responsibility or authority for departmental management or governance decisions.

"What Attracts Potential Donors?"

Since most donors consider their gifts as investments, they are attracted to activities they value and leaders they trust. Their assessment usually includes past success, future plans, and the availability of additional resources to ensure the sustainability and desired impact of their gift. In addition, most donors are interested in your record of tracking and ensuring the accomplishments and outcomes of donations. In this regard, many donors consider their contributions more like contracts with timed deliverables rather than unrestricted gifts or grants.

Stewardship of gifts is essential to ensure donor satisfaction. Regular progress reports (at least annually) along with social interactions (e.g., luncheons) go far in keeping donors satisfied. If the donor has named a scholarship, fellowship, or an endowed chair, you should have the recipients meet with the donor on a recurring basis to help maintain their satisfaction and assure them that their investment is worthwhile. Hearing directly from the individuals who benefit from their gifts also can increase their potential interest in providing additional donations.

As noted above, many donors wish to have their gift named. It is useful for your relationship with donors to proactively suggest that their name or that of a loved one or mentor be associated with the donation to provide appropriate recognition. Such naming also can help your development activities by making donations visible to other potential donors. It is useful to have examples of prior donations available to show a potential donor the nature and scope of the contributions that others have made. This can help assure the donor that others are supportive of your programs, suggesting that their own investments in the department will be safe and impactful.

"What Do Potential Donors Worry About?"

In addition to the fear that their donation may have little impact, a major concern of most donors is that the intended use of their gift is not being met. Unfortunately, it is not uncommon that a large contribution to a program is accompanied by some reduction in departmental or institutional support for that program in order to free up funds for other priorities. Diverting donations to cover other activities and reducing departmental support for programs receiving donations should be avoided but, if done, should be made transparent in order to ensure the donor's trust.

A related concern of donors is that the use of their endowment will change after their death. The best way to assure donors that you, your department, and the institution are committed to their intent is by prior example. Ongoing use of the endowment can also be part of the written gift agreement as long as there is departmental or institutional support for such. Contingency funding should also be explicit for cases where the program that is endowed may end (e.g., a degree or research program, department subsection).

Donors also may be concerned that the activities they support in your department will not be successful. When educating donors, it is important to focus on the opportunities that additional support could provide, rather than about programs being under-funded, which implies that they may be unsuccessful or a low priority for the institution; donors want to invest in success and high priority areas.

Active communication and ongoing follow-up with donors about the use and impact of their gifts are critically important for stewarding the relationship. Donors should be made to feel that they have a special connection with the department and institution, as well as the leaders with whom they have been involved. Being transparent with donors about the use of their gifts is critical to maintaining a trusting relationship. A breach of trust with any donor is likely to become known by other donors as well as institutional leaders, which can have detrimental effects with spiraling consequences beyond fundraising, especially for you personally.

"Whom Should I Try to Develop as Donors to My Department?"

There are several categories of potential donors for you to consider including grateful patients, community leaders, alumni (students, trainees, faculty, staff), and especially prior donors [2]. You should work with your institutional development office(s) to help identify specific individuals in these categories whom you could consider developing as potential donors, especially during a fundraising campaign.

Most AHCs/AMCs have a grateful patient program to identify and engage patients who are potential donors. Key contacts for these programs are the medical staff involved in providing care to the potential donor. These programs vary widely, and some are primarily hospital or medical school based rather than departmentally focused; in any case you should make sure that you and your department are active participants and follow institutional guidelines for all interactions.

Because of the local importance of AHCs/AMCs, members of the community are often interested in contributing to its success. Such potential donors may be interested in helping the community by supporting local clinical service programs or more broadly by funding research, education, or outreach initiatives. Providing community education programs can help stimulate local donor interest in your department's activities. In addition to creating a community "Board of Visitors/ Advisors" as mentioned above, departmental open houses with presentations by clinical and research faculty may also stimulate interest in funding.

Alumni students, trainees, faculty, and staff who greatly benefitted from their previous time in your department usually have a strong commitment to its ongoing success and should be actively engaged as potential donors. Their experience and understanding often results in their gratitude being focused on supporting a specific area of familiarity in your department. This often requires less time for you to update them about the department and its programs, but more time to develop their confidence, especially if you are new to the department.

As previously noted, it is well accepted that your best potential donors are your past donors. Past donors have already shown their interest in supporting your initiatives and, if they have been stewarded appropriately, often will follow an initial gift with a larger one.

"How Do I Deal with Conflicts Over Donors with Whom Other Departments or the Institution Are Engaging?"

In many cases, potential donors have an interest or relationship with other programs and individuals at your AHC/AMC, as well as your parent and affiliated institutions. This can create conflicts within the institution and also for the donor. You should determine if your institution(s) has formal "rules of engagement" with past and active donors and clearance processes for approaching them. This is especially important if you have more than one parent or affiliated institution with separate development staffs.

Before engaging a potential donor who already has a relationship with the institution, you always should check with your development leadership team(s) to be sure you are not in conflict with other development activities that may be in progress. Being transparent and collaborative in the fundraising process at your institution(s) is an important part of being considered a team player.

In many cases the interests of a donor span two or more departments, programs, or institutions. Depending on the processes and rules at your institution(s), you may need to take a back seat in dealing with such donors or in some cases be asked to take the lead. Losing a potential donor because they feel pulled in different directions is a major failure for all concerned. Avoiding potential conflicts in donor interactions is in your best interest as well as that of your institution(s) and the donor.

In contrast to the problems that can be created by multiple independent and conflicting contacts with a donor, there are substantial benefits in coordinated fundraising activities among multiple institutional leaders and programs. The importance of having the development staffs of departments and institutions coordinated and working together when engaging a donor cannot be over-emphasized. A coherent, consistent interaction sends a powerful message about the alignment of interests among the leaders and programs that are involved, and projects a strong predictor of success for the donor. Joint fundraising across departments, programs, and especially academic and health-care institutions is synergistic and worth developing whenever possible. Areas particularly attractive to donors and well positioned for joint fundraising include interdisciplinary programs mentioned above (i.e., cancer, heart disease, children's health, infectious diseases, informatics, and genetics).

Dealing with Foundations

"How Do I Deal with Foundations?"

Fundraising often involves interactions with foundations, either as an entity that executes a donor's commitment or as the initial point of contact leading to an interaction with foundation staff. In either case, it is important to understand the foundation's priorities, processes, and organizational model. In particular, learning how their approval process works and who ultimately makes decisions can help focus your time and effort.

When a foundation benefactor is still actively engaged, the foundation board often acts to simply advise, and contributions are effectively decided by the benefactor. In cases where the benefactor is not engaged or has died, and the foundation board makes funding decisions, you should learn who on the board and administrative team are the important contacts to engage in your development activities. Be sure to involve your institutional development team when working with foundations for the information they can provide and to avoid conflicts.

An important consideration when engaging foundations is to determine whether the time and effort is worth the opportunity costs involved. Some foundations require significant effort in their funding process for relatively small grants or a low chance of success. Here again, getting input from your development office and peers who previously have engaged with a foundation is well advised.

Creating a Development Program for Your Department

"How Do I Build a Successful Departmental Development Program?"

The keys to establishing a successful development program for your department are to be well aligned with your institutional development activity and to have your faculty well educated and engaged. Your first step should be to work with your institutional development office(s) to understand the rules and processes for fundraising and developing donors at your institution(s) [3–5].

Staffing for development activity at most AHCs/AMCs is centralized, with development officers assigned to specific departments and programs. Depending on your department's size and potential, the development staff assigned may be shared among multiple units. Funding for development officers may also be centralized, with the option for units to directly fund additional development staff.

When staffing is centralized, there often is tension among departments over the support they are provided. Staff distribution is usually based on past success and future potential of fundraising, so if you feel that your department is under-staffed, be sure to evaluate these parameters before requesting additional development support or investing your own departmental funds. You should also evaluate past and potential financial return on your direct and indirect departmental expenses for fundraising to determine how much to allocate for future development activities in the context of your strategic plan and budget. The indirect costs in faculty/staff time and effort for fundraising can be substantial and easily underestimated.

Although development staff support is important, the principal factor for successful fundraising is the engagement of your faculty. As discussed above, donors and foundations make contributions to people and programs they value and believe will be successful, and their confidence and trust in the faculty leading these activities is paramount. In addition, donors often develop significant relationships with departmental as well as fundraising staff to shepherd their access and interactions. It is well-worth the effort to educate your faculty and staff on how best to develop and interact with donors, which can be done with appropriate development officers or by bringing in outside experts. The importance you place on development and its potential benefits for faculty programs will help stimulate them to engage in fundraising.

It also is beneficial to engage students and trainees in your fundraising and development activities. They can be very effective in soliciting gifts by phone for general programs (e.g., discretionary annual funds), as well as specific programs (e.g., scholarships, fellowships), especially for activities in which they are involved personally. If you have donors who have provided endowed scholarships or fellowships, it is important to create opportunities for them to meet with recipients. This allows them to see and hear first-hand how their gifts are benefiting specific individuals, which often encourages them to make additional contributions.

"How Much of My Own Time Should I Allocate to Fundraising and Donor Development?"

Fundraising and donor development can take a tremendous amount of your time and effort. In addition to the programs and donors of your own personal interest, faculty and development officers will often want you to engage with donors that are being developed, and many donors will want to meet you as the department chair. Part of educating your faculty about fundraising is to have them understand your personal priorities for helping with their development activities. Factors you should consider for how much time to spend on development activities and with specific donors include the potential amount of a contribution, the importance of the donor, and the priority of the program being funded.

References

1. Bailey DN, Crawford JM, Jensen PE, Leonard DGB, McCarthy S, Sanfilippo F. Generating discretionary income in an academic department of pathology. Acad Pathol. 2021;8:23742895211044811. https://doi.org/10.1177/23742895211044811.
2. Winstead DK. Advice for chairs of academic departments of psychiatry: the "ten commandments". Acad Psychiatry. 2006;30:298–300. https://doi.org/10.1176/appi.ap.30.4.298.
3. Brody WR, Fishman EK, Chu LC, Rowe SP. Brother, can you spare a dime? An introduction to philanthropy and fundraising. J Am Coll Radiol. 2021;18:1466–8. https://doi.org/10.1016/j.jacr.2021.04.003.
4. Buller JL. The essential department chair: a comprehensive desk reference. 2nd ed. San Francisco, CA: Jossey-Bass; 2012. ISBN 978-1118123744.
5. Mallon WT, Grigsby RK. Leading: top skills, attributes, and behaviors critical for success. Washington, DC: Association of American Medical Colleges; 2016. ISBN 978-1577541509.

Part VIII
Personal Issues

Developing the skills and knowledge to become a good leader involves time, effort, and experience and is greatly enhanced by the advice and assistance you can get from others. The motivation needed to improve as a leader requires good self-awareness, an understanding of what you don't know, and the ability to deal with criticism. Advisors, mentors, and coaches can help your leadership development along with the feedback you receive from performance reviews of you and your department. Work-life balance and wellness are critical to your success as a leader, to both strengthen your resilience and performance and serve as a role model for your faculty, staff, students, and trainees. Knowing when to consider transitioning to another position and evaluating potential options are issues you must face at some point. While stressful, career transitions can be exhilarating and provide new opportunities for your professional development and personal satisfaction.

Chapter 33
Leadership Attributes

Characteristics of Successful Leaders

"Why Should I Want to Be a Department Chair?"

Great leaders seek their position not because of its stature or title, but because they wish to accomplish something important for their organization and its members. At the outset of your position, you should determine what you want to accomplish as a leader, be sure that it is consistent with institutional expectations, and estimate the timeline and relative priorities needed for achieving these goals.

You should view your leadership role as a privilege to serve your institution and your department and be focused on how you can improve the performance and success of your faculty, staff, and students, rather than feeling that you are the boss and can exert control over people and resources. Great leaders have the simple mindset that they are working for others, and not that others are working for them.

"What Are the Behaviors, Skills, and Style of Successful Leaders?"

To be a successful leader you should strive to be:

- *Altruistic*, placing the interests of the department and institution above your own
- *Decisive*, making informed decisions after collecting all pertinent information
- *Collegial*, always willing to give help and advice as needed
- *Committed*, truly dedicated to the success of your team, department, and institution
- *Compassionate*, helping those needing advice or assistance
- *Confident*, knowing your strengths and weaknesses

© The Author(s), under exclusive license to Springer Nature Switzerland AG 2023

F. Sanfilippo et al., *Lead, Inspire, Thrive*, https://doi.org/10.1007/978-3-031-41177-9_33

- *Constructive*, providing advice and criticism in a helpful manner
- *Courageous*, unafraid to take an unpopular stand for a good reason or cause
- *Empathic*, caring about the welfare and success of your faculty, staff, students, trainees, and colleagues
- *Entrepreneurial*, willing to take well-informed, well-intentioned risks
- *Fair*, treating everyone the same without regard to their respective positions
- *Flexible*, handling new and different situations with ease
- *Future-oriented*, guiding long-term success by anticipating and adapting to change
- *Honest*, refusing to be deceitful
- *Humble*, not focused on self-promotion and always willing to give others credit
- *Influential*, providing valuable thoughts and ideas to others
- *Innovative*, being creative and leading in new ways and in new directions
- *Inquisitive*, looking for new ideas, advice, and input
- *Inspirational*, stimulating others to be encouraged and productive
- *Integrity*, having strong principles and doing the right thing
- *Knowledgeable*, of what you know and do not know
- *Observant*, paying attention to people and situations
- *Open-minded*, soliciting and considering all viewpoints on issues
- *Optimistic*, inspiring members of your department and serving as a positive role model
- *Passionate*, focused on achieving the expectations set for you and your department
- *Proactive*, being ahead of issues and opportunities rather than reacting to them
- *Responsible*, being accountable and fulfilling the duties of your position
- *Resilient*, being able to deal with the stress and pressures of your leadership position
- *Self-aware*, understanding your strengths, weaknesses, motivations, and behavior
- *Transparent*, sharing nonconfidential information used to make decisions
- *Trustworthy*, honoring all agreements and promises
- *Visionary*, able to forecast trends and to lead your department into the future

Furthermore, to be a successful leader you should strive to:

- Become an excellent communicator, knowing how to clearly articulate your thoughts and ideas and appreciating the expectations of your audience (see Chap. 5).
- Lead by example and never ask someone to do something unless you are willing to do it yourself [1].
- Not be afraid to make well-informed, well-intentioned mistakes and learn from them and the mistakes made by others.
- Accept responsibility when things go wrong and apologize sincerely [1].
- Follow the chain of command laid out by institutional leaders and institutional organization charts.
- Be organized and an expert at time management, maintaining control of your schedules and not allowing yourself to be overscheduled (see Chap. 36, section "Time Management at Work").

- Maintain confidentiality and not speak disparagingly of other faculty, staff, administrators, or institutional leaders.
- Have a team mentality, providing them support and seeking their advice and feedback continually.
- Document agreements in writing and summarize the outcome of important meetings.
- Have personal role models who continue to inspire you.
- Develop a proper work-life balance, realizing that refreshing yourself is good not only for you but also for the department (see Chap. 36).

"How Do I Lead in the Rapidly Changing World of Academic Medicine?"

This is a time of unprecedented change in academic medicine. New models of health-care delivery (especially telehealth and the use of chatbots), as well as changing reimbursements, increased attention to social determinants of health, and an overdue imperative to address health disparities will shape the future clinical mission. Breakthrough advances in science and technology, gene manipulation, the development of AI (artificial intelligence) algorithms and applications, and increased understanding of cellular and molecular mechanism are refocusing the research mission. New pedagogy, innovative digital approaches to learning, and the changing demographics of trainees demand new approaches to the educational mission. And new challenges from pandemics to racial injustice to climate change and more impact our AMCs/AHCs and those they serve. In light of this, chairs must not only manage and lead successfully in the current environment, but also guide their department to be positioned for success in the coming decades and beyond [2].

The need for chairs to be "future-oriented" has been a clarion call for years and remains a critical goal [3, 4]. A future-oriented leader must not only personally embrace change, but also inspire others to be excited about the new possibilities. This requires chairs to create safe spaces that encourage innovation and change evaluation procedures to avoid discouraging risk-taking by punishing failure. As a chair who needs to prepare for an uncertain future, you should openly and authentically acknowledge the known and unknown challenges, and encourage all stakeholders to join you in envisioning the importance, excitement, and satisfaction of solving problems in academic medicine and in defining new paths that improve all those impacted by your work. Openness to new ideas, enthusiasm for trying new programs and approaches, willingness to take appropriate risks, evaluation of innovations, and resilience and persistence in responding to new challenges and opportunities will be key to your future success.

Evaluation of Leadership Skills

"How Do I Know If I Have the Skills of a Successful Leader?"

Most leaders will know their relative success (or failure) as a leader from the formal and informal feedback they receive from members of their department, peers, and especially the institutional leaders to whom they report. Most leadership positions require reviews of achievements and meeting expectations on a regular basis, e.g., annually and at the end of the leadership term (see Chap. 35). These reviews usually include an assessment of leadership skills and may involve a 360° evaluation by the circle of individuals who work with the leader.

Developing and Maintaining Self-Awareness

"How Do I Become More Self-Aware of My Own Strengths and Weaknesses?"

Self-awareness involves understanding your strengths, weaknesses, motivations, and character traits and how they affect your thoughts and behavior. Self-awareness is often considered one of the most important attributes of good leaders because it impacts so many other aspects of leadership, as detailed above. The key to developing and maintaining self-awareness is getting frequent feedback from others about your strengths, weaknesses, behavior, and character. To do this, let your faculty, staff, leadership team, institutional peers, and colleagues know that you truly desire candid feedback, and that comments about your weaknesses and negative behavior would be especially appreciated.

Unfortunately, many faculty and staff in your department, including members of your leadership team, may be reluctant to provide you with candid input about your weaknesses or negative behavioral and character traits. When asked for input, they may not want to appear critical and will primarily focus on your strengths, which can provide you with a misleading view of your behavior and leadership. As mentioned in Chap. 11 (see section "Building Your Team"), it is important to have some key lieutenants who are highly trusted by faculty and staff to act as intermediaries to get candid feedback. Inputs from faculty and staff through these lieutenants, as well as their own feedback, are invaluable ways to develop and maintain awareness of your strengths, weaknesses, and behavior.

Other important sources of input are institutional peers with whom you have a close relationship and who have interactions with your department, as well as your peers at other institutions who likewise may have contacts with members of your department. Feedback from your supervisor(s) when they perform the annual review of your leadership performance can be very helpful in identifying your strengths and weaknesses, as can the detailed feedback from departmental reviews (see Chap. 35). The use of a 360° review can be extremely helpful in providing input from department faculty and staff, institutional peers, and leaders in a comprehensive, standardized manner [5]. As discussed in the next chapter, input from advisors, mentors, and coaches also can help you increase your self-awareness.

"How Should I Deal with Mistakes?"

Remember, no one is perfect. Mistakes can be minimized by asking for advice (see Chap. 34), listening carefully, and making thoughtful decisions. But when you do make mistakes (and you will), be transparent and address them quickly and forthrightly. Try not to punish yourself for mistakes; an important attribute of resilience is realizing that everyone makes mistakes and, when well-intended, you should have self-compassion when they occur. Showing humility rather than making excuses will be appreciated by those around you, and owning up to your mistakes will serve as an important role model for other departmental faculty, staff, students, trainees, and leaders when they make mistakes.

Leadership Training

"Where Can I Obtain Formal Leadership Training?"

Just as with any other skill you wish to develop and improve, good training is important to improve your ability as a good leader. Your daily activities as a leader can provide many opportunities to learn how to be a better leader, especially if you spend some time focusing on improving your leadership skills. In addition, formal leadership training is available from many sources and in many formats.

Most academic institutions have formal leadership training programs for their new faculty leaders and for those aspiring to be leaders [6]. These usually can be accessed through your institutional offices of faculty affairs and HR. Many require completing a capstone project, and a number of them offer a certificate upon completion of the curriculum. If your AHC/AMC does not offer such programs, several institutions offer them to those who are not on their faculty such as the Harvard Executive Leadership Program (HELP) and the Drexel University Executive Leadership in Academic Medicine (ELAM) Program.

Many professional societies also offer leadership development programs and you should consult the professional organizations in your discipline to find such programs. In addition, leadership training at a wide range of levels is available from several organizations including the AAMC [7], the AHA [8], the Center for Creative Leadership [9], and the Chronicle of Higher Education Strategic Leadership

Program for Department Chairs [10]. As mentioned in Chap. 18 (section "Resources for Career Development"), most business schools have executive education courses and programs for enhancing leadership skills in specific areas (e.g., negotiation, finance, communication, strategy, management, and more).

Leadership programs also can be augmented by coaches, advisors, and mentors who can help you understand and develop leadership attributes (see Chap. 34). Coaches can enhance your leadership skills through training experience, while advisors can help you deal with specific leadership issues. Mentors also can provide long-term evaluation and help in guiding the leadership aspects of your career.

Dealing with Criticism

"How Should I Handle Criticism?"

An inevitable part of leadership is receiving criticism. Criticism can come at any time from any source and often is completely unanticipated. As a department chair, you should expect that not all of your faculty and staff will agree with every decision you make, and that some institutional peers, leaders, and other stakeholders may question or be disappointed in some of your actions. Any of these disagreements or disappointments can result in criticism directed at you personally. How you respond can have a significant impact on your subsequent job performance, satisfaction, and well-being.

Over-reacting to criticism can be counter-productive by precipitating a serious conflict that destroys your relationship with the critic. Moreover, over-reacting aggressively or defensively will be viewed by some as inappropriate and representing a character flaw. For you personally, it can become a significant distraction and cause unneeded additional stress in your life. As much as possible, you should simply accept that receiving criticism is part of the job, regardless of how hard you try to do the right thing as a leader. And, as with making mistakes, you should strengthen your resilience with self-compassion.

The best way to respond to criticism is objectively and dispassionately. Evaluate the criticism at face value and resist considering it a personal attack, even if it is. Don't become distracted by trying to determine an underlying intent. Rather, respond directly to the specific points raised with facts and data, and appreciate that criticism often contains a useful point of view and information that might be constructive. It often helps to evaluate criticism by taking the critic's position, which can make it easier to find some value in the criticism and avoid an emotional reaction. If an aspect of the criticism appears appropriate, demonstrate humility and acknowledge that you have made a mistake and are grateful for the feedback.

If the criticism is without merit and simply meant as a personal attack, it becomes even more important to respond dispassionately and objectively with facts. Showing anger or emotion, especially when others are present, will help an inappropriate critic accomplish their goal, so avoid behavior and body language that suggest you have been hurt personally. Taking the high road and not being dismissive or launching a counter-attack will be recognized by most as a strength rather than a weakness and will provide a positive role model for others.

Handling Conflicts of Interest

"How Should I Handle Conflicts of Interest?"

Conflicts of interest are of many types and can occur in each mission area, e.g., having stock options in a company that is funding one's research, using a trainee to work on a project that provides personal benefits, and referring patients to an enterprise in which one has a financial interest. They also may involve personal relationships, such as completing a performance evaluation of a friend or hiring someone who is related to you. In general, any situation that provides, or appears to provide, a personal benefit to you or your immediate family members could involve a conflict of interest. As a leader, you should be constantly alert to both real and perceived conflicts of interest, since you will be held responsible for those involving your faculty as well as yourself.

Conflicts of interests often cannot be resolved completely, but you should know the processes for managing them. As is often said, "no conflict, no interest." For financial conflicts of interest, there are many regulations requiring disclosure of the potential conflicts. Most institutions have a process that requires full disclosure of financial and other potential conflicts, which are reviewed and determined to be allowed, disallowed, or managed in a specific manner.

Federal funding agencies including the National Institutes of Health (NIH), National Science Foundation (NSF), Department of Energy (DOE), Department of Defense (DOD), as well as most foundations and state funding agencies mandate disclosures of potential financial conflicts of interest by grant and contract recipients, as do for-profit companies and non-profit organizations that provide support. These potential conflicts also apply if the spouse or partner of the funding recipient has the conflict.

Mitigation strategies may include issuing a "best practices memo" requiring the recipient to disclose the potential conflict in any publications and talks, and having an internal review committee monitor the conflict to ensure compliance with and necessary disclosures. For nonfinancial conflicts, it is equally incumbent upon you and your faculty to be forthcoming with disclosures.

Most organizations also have regulations precluding supervision of one's family members and voting on issues involving the welfare/well-being of an individual close to you. Most institutions have conflict of interest and risk management offices and officers that can offer advice, and you should use them without hesitation.

Failure to disclose conflicts can irreparably damage one's career and lead to loss of one's leadership position. A simple rule of thumb is to be concerned if you even *wonder* if a situation may represent a conflict of interest. It is better to disclose when it may not be necessary than fail to disclose when it is required.

Maintaining Confidentiality

"How Do I Know What to Keep Confidential and What I May Disclose?"

While you should strive to be transparent whenever possible, you must resist any temptation to disclose information given to you in confidence. You should realize that not all individuals will convey confidential information to you with the *proviso* that you should keep the information confidential. Unless explicitly told by the confider that you may share the information with anyone, or it is already in the public domain, you should assume that it is confidential, particularly if it involves an individual's personal life situation or an individual's relationship with co-workers. Ask yourself "if I were that individual would I want that information disclosed?" Also, you should assume that many confidential matters are press-worthy, and consider the consequences if information you divulge ends up in the media. Ask yourself "would I want to see this information in my local newspaper?"

Exceptions to the above policy include disclosure of information for the common good (e.g., someone's threat to commit a crime) and disclosure of a violation of a legal rule or policy that you are required to report as an institutional leader (e.g., sexual harassment or abuse, an accusation of research misconduct). If you anticipate that someone is about to disclose a matter that you are required to report, you may preempt the disclosure and refer the individual to the appropriate institutional officer. Some activities may require a nondisclosure agreement, which legally binds the individual from disclosing information that would potentially harm the other party.

In the instance of research misconduct, most institutions have formal processes for investigation under the auspices of their Office of Research Integrity. In cases involving sexual harassment, Title IX violations, and other instances of discrimination based on gender, sexual orientation, disability, age, race, and ethnicity, you should contact your appropriate institutional office.

References

1. Gilbert FJ. Ten lessons of leadership: reflections of a female academic. Clin Radiol. 2020;75:799–803. https://doi.org/10.1016/j.crad.2020.07.005.

2. Salazar D, Herndon JH, Vail TP, Zuckerman JD, Gelberman RH. The academic chair: achieving success in a rapidly-evolving health-care environment: AOA critical issues. J Bone Joint Surg Am. 2018;100:e133. https://doi.org/10.2106/JBJS.17.01056.
3. Bras RL, DeMillo RA. The leadership challenges for higher education's digital future. In: Antony JS, Cauce AM, Shalala DE, editors. Challenges in higher education leadership. Routledge; 2017. p. 39–56. ISBN 978-1138884878.
4. Grigsby RK, Hefner DS, Souba WW, Kirch DG. The future-oriented department chair. Acad Med. 2004;79:571–7. https://doi.org/10.1097/00001888-200406000-00014.
5. Hu J, Lee R, Mullin S, Schwaitzberg S, Harmon L, Gregory P, et al. How physicians change: multisource feedback driven intervention improves physician leadership and teamwork. Surgery. 2020;168(4):714–23. https://doi.org/10.1016/j.surg.2020.06.008.
6. Lucas RL, Goldman EF, Scott AR, Dandar V. Leadership development programs at academic health centers: results of a national survey. Acad Med. 2018;93:229–36. https://doi.org/10.1097/ACM.0000000000001813.
7. Association of American Medical Colleges. https://www.aamc.org/career-development/leadership-development.
8. American Hospital Association. https://www.aha.org/center/next-generation-leaders-fellowship.
9. Center for Creative Leadership. https://www.ccl.org/leadership-challenges/executive-leadership-programs/.
10. Chronicle of Higher Education: The chronicle's strategic-leadership program: department chairs. https://www.chronicle.com/professional-development/events/the-chronicles-strategic-leadership-program-department-chairs?cid=gen_sign_in. Accessed 21 Oct 2022.

Chapter 34
Getting Advice and Assistance

Advisors and Consultants

"When Should I Use an Advisor or a Consultant?"

It often becomes apparent that you need advice or help to adequately address a specific problem or opportunity. Advisors have experience in dealing with the decisions you are facing and help by providing recommendations and new ideas. Getting input and suggestions from advisors is useful for issues that are complex or outside the experience and comfort level of you and your team, especially involving people, process, and technical matters. Given the personal association advisors frequently have with their advisees, they usually do not charge for their advice.

In contrast, consultants are professionals who charge for their services to assist you in getting work done. Engaging a consultant is helpful when you and your team do not have the time, expertise, or staff available to appropriately deal with an issue. Assistance from a consultant can include supplying temporary personnel with specific skills to work on a project, supporting strategic and tactical initiatives, and providing options and potential outcomes for using or obtaining resources, especially space, equipment, and personnel. Consultants can also be helpful to you in making challenging decisions (e.g., cutting personnel budgets), since they provide external objective perspectives that are often better accepted by the leaders to whom you report, members of your department, and other stakeholders. When using consultants, you should ensure that the work product desired is explicitly described in the contract.

F. Sanfilippo et al., *Lead, Inspire, Thrive*,
https://doi.org/10.1007/978-3-031-41177-9_34

"How Do I Find the Right Advisor or Consultant to Help Me with a Specific Issue?"

Advisors are often peers whom you know through a professional, institutional, or prior relationship. Most colleagues are glad to help others with advice from their personal experience. When seeking advice, you should look for someone you respect and trust with expertise and experience in dealing with the issue at hand. If appropriate, your predecessor might have a good understanding of the issues you face and could be a valuable source for advice (see Chap. 4, section "Advice and Assistance"). Also, former department chairs in your discipline (either at your institution or elsewhere) may be excellent sources for advice [1].

The ability to keep an issue and the advice you get confidential is often an important factor in finding the right advisor, especially for personal matters. In situations when an advisor is not readily apparent for a particular subject, ask peers you trust whom they might recommend.

To find the right consultant for helping with a specific need, you should evaluate professional, consumer-oriented individuals and companies that have a well-documented track record in the area requiring assistance. Although searching for the right consultant has become easier with the wealth of information available online and through social media, it is always wise to get a personal recommendation from a prior client before finalizing a consulting agreement.

When deciding whether to solicit help from an advisor or consultant there are several things to consider:

- *Issues*: for issues simply requiring recommendations and guidance, an advisor is normally sufficient. For issues requiring assistance with detailed assessments, planning, and/or implementation, a consultant is needed.
- *Complexity*: for issues with multiple components and significant intricacy, a consultant team is usually needed to provide the depth and breadth of support required for evaluation and resolution.
- *Timeframe*: for issues requiring resolution quickly, an advisor can usually help without needing to develop deliverables and a contract, which would take additional time with a consultant. For issues having a specific due date, an explicit contract agreement with a consultant may provide greater assurance of completing the work on time.
- *Cost*: an advisor usually will not charge you, while consultants will require payment and a contract for their anticipated work product and deliverables.

In evaluating potential advisors or consultants, it is useful to clearly delineate the most important goals for getting the advice or assistance to be sure it corresponds with their expertise. In addition, you should appreciate that every advisor or consultant has particular strengths, weaknesses, and biases in how they approach, evaluate, and provide advice or assistance, so make sure their behavior and culture are an appropriate match for you and your team.

Mentors

"How Should I Find and Develop a Relationship with a Mentor?"

Mentors are trusted counselors who establish a strong, personal, and long-term relationship with individuals to help guide them, especially in their career planning and development. Most leaders find mentors throughout their career, beginning with teachers who provided career counseling and a special relationship. Subsequently, mentors often can be solicited from supervisors and senior members in the profession or institution who are interested in the career development of the individual. Given their personal, long-term relationship, mentors do not charge for their services.

Chairs and other leaders often have several mentors with whom they have developed relationships over the years. The use of several mentors can provide you with different perspectives and viewpoints [2]. In follow-up to your recruitment, the chair or a member of the search committee will sometimes offer or can be asked to provide mentorship. Professional societies also will often have senior members in the field who can be approached as mentors [3]. Receiving advice and counsel from mentors is a precious gift that should be highly appreciated and reciprocated by your willingness to mentor others.

Coaches

"When Do I Need Coaching?"

Coaches are instructors who help improve the performance of those they teach and train. A great lesson for leaders who don't think they need coaching is the fact that the best athletes in the world use coaches extensively to help improve their performance. Moreover, there is substantial evidence that good coaching is a critical part of a leader's performance [4, 5]. Essentially all leaders can benefit from coaching to strengthen areas of weakness and enhance areas of strength.

Leadership coaching can be focused on several different behavioral attributes and performance skills. In particular, it can help you develop more constructive behaviors and better engage your faculty and institutional leadership, which in turn can result in improved overall performance and satisfaction. Another benefit of good leadership coaching is to increase your self-awareness, which is a critical attribute that is often diminished or skewed as one moves into higher leadership positions (see Chap. 33, section "Developing and Maintaining Self-Awareness")".

"How Do I Find the Right Coach for Me?"

The first step in finding the right coach is to get a comprehensive assessment to determine the strengths and weaknesses of your personal leadership behaviors and style (see Chap. 33). This will reveal the areas for you to work on and help identify what type of coaching would be most beneficial. Since coaches must be constructive critics to help you see and then work on areas needing improvement, it is important to find a coach whose temperament and approach are ones you can respond to positively. Since coaches are paid professionals, the criteria for selecting them are similar in many respects to the approach discussed above for selecting a consultant. However, a coach is more like a mentor in regard to developing a long-term personal relationship with a focus on your personal performance and success.

Sponsors

"What Is a Sponsor and How Can I Find an Appropriate One?"

At various points in your career you may want to be nominated for awards, prizes, and membership in prestigious societies and seek references for certain positions. Accordingly, it is important for you to cultivate relationships with individuals who can sponsor you for such opportunities. An advisor or mentor often will be the most appropriate, but colleagues and acquaintances may be very useful as sponsors, especially based on their relationship to the organization offering the award or position.

If a sponsor is eager and willing to nominate/endorse you when asked, you should make the process as easy as possible for them. Also, be sure to express your gratitude for their help, describe the potential impact it may have on your career, and keep them appraised of the follow-up. If a potential sponsor does not appear to be enthusiastic about a particular award or position, avoid bothering them, but don't necessarily rule them out for a subsequent request that they might feel is more appropriate. Once a sponsor has supported you, you should stay in touch with them so that you can use them for future reference.

Family and Friends

"When Should I Ask Family and Friends for Advice?"

Family and friends are an important source of advice and assistance because of their trust, candor, and interest in your personal success and satisfaction. This is often a good counter-balance to the advice of others who may have more experience or expertise about the issues being considered, but do not have as deep an understanding of your personality and values.

Clearly, personal issues such as career choices, self-awareness, and work-life balance should always be discussed with family and trusted friends, and it is often helpful to ask their advice about job-related issues as well. However, candid conversations about job-related individuals and activities should be carefully tempered with the understanding that such work-related issues are confidential and must remain so, unless directly impacting decisions in your personal life, such as career transitions (see Chap. 37, section "Knowing When It's Time").

Having to describe an issue to someone outside their area of expertise can be extremely helpful by exposing aspects that may not have been appreciated by others who may be looking at too many of the details and not the bigger picture. Moreover, the better appreciation by family and friends of your personality, behavior, and body language in a more candid discussion might reveal subjective aspects not appreciated by advisors, consultants, or mentors. Some of the best thought-provoking questions that generate new ideas about an issue may come from those who least understand the details.

References

1. Bailey DN, Cohen S, Gotlieb A, Lipscomb MF, Sanfilippo F. What advice current pathology chairs seek from former chairs. Acad Pathol. 2018;5:2374289518807397. https://doi.org/10.1177/2374289518807397.
2. Khatchikian AD, Chahal BS, Kielar A. Mosaic mentoring: finding the right mentor for the issue at hand. Abdom Radiol. 2021;46:5480–4. https://doi.org/10.1007/s00261-021-03314-2.
3. Sanfilippo F, Markwood P, Bailey DN. Retaining the value of former department chairs: the association of pathology chairs experience. Acad Pathol. 2020;7:2374289520981685. https://doi.org/10.1177/2374289520981685.
4. Anthony EL. The impact of leadership coaching on leadership behaviors. J Manag Dev. 2017;36:930–9. https://doi.org/10.1108/JMD-06-2016-0092.
5. Gawande A. Personal best. Ann Med. 2011. https://www.newyorker.com/magazine/2011/10/03/personal-best. Accessed 27 Aug 2022.

Chapter 35
Handling Reviews

Dealing with Personal Reviews

"How Should I Approach My Annual Review?"

Essentially all institutions require an annual appraisal of employees including department chairs and other leaders, to provide feedback on the past year's performance and expectations for the next year. You should always use these reviews as a valuable way to get input on the performance of you and your department, and especially about potential opportunities to help the institution [1].

In most cases you will be asked to submit a written report on your progress and that of your department over the past year, in which you should focus on the expectations that were delineated in previous reviews as well as at the onset of your tenure as chair. Emphasis should be made on how your department has helped the institution in its mission, priorities, and goals. Your leadership team should help put the report together, and it is wise to have it reviewed by trusted advisors and colleagues before submission. The report should be candid and shared with the department as appropriate.

Because your institutional leaders likely have many department chairs reporting to them, these annual reviews are often performed by one of their surrogates. Listen carefully during your review and ask questions to make sure you understand what is being said. Avoid responding too quickly or strongly to any negative statements about your past performance or future expectations with which you disagree. In such cases, ask for more details and especially a written summary so you can clearly understand the deficient performance issues or disagreeable expectations that are provided, and respond that you will follow up after you can process the information. This will give you the opportunity to develop a thoughtful response, which you should discuss with your trusted advisors.

F. Sanfilippo et al., *Lead, Inspire, Thrive*,
https://doi.org/10.1007/978-3-031-41177-9_35

If your reviewer was a surrogate for the leader(s) to whom you report, do not bypass your reviewer to follow up with your boss(es) first; this will be viewed as an end-around and hurt your relationship with both your reviewer and your boss(es). Try to resolve any disagreements with your actual reviewer before bringing them to the next-level leaders.

"How Should I Respond to Personal Recommendations in My Department Review?"

As discussed below, most department reviews will evaluate how well chairs have performed in leading their department to achieve its goals and expectations, and, as appropriate, provide priorities and goals for the chair as well as the department. If your department review is at the end of your current term and you are interested in continuing, a recommendation usually will be provided regarding your reappointment, which may be for a limited term if some remediation is needed. Your personal evaluation normally would not be discussed during your meeting with the review committee, but provided directly to institutional leadership. Your institutional leaders may discuss this aspect of the review with you before the written report is received, or choose to wait for the written report to discuss its findings and present follow-up plans.

If you disagree with some of the review findings or your leadership's expectations, you should avoid the temptation to respond immediately. Take time to assess the information provided and get advice from trusted mentors and other advisors (see Chap. 34). Carefully consider possible responses, and especially potential consequences, before responding to leadership.

"How Should I Handle a Targeted Review of My Performance or Behavior?"

Reviews conducted to only assess a specific performance or behavioral issue of a chair are rare and may include some components of a department evaluation (see below). If a review is focused on your personal performance rather than on the department, you should obtain a clear understanding of the rationale, purpose, scope, process, and confidentiality of the review from your leadership beforehand, and discuss any concerns you may have. In particular, if you feel such a review involves an unfair process, is not about your performance or behavior, or is inappropriate (e.g., a personal attack following a disagreement), you should consider getting legal advice to protect yourself. Be sure to document correspondence and take notes during meetings. Remember that the simple act of leadership initiating a targeted personal review can have a significant negative impact on your reputation.

You may consider avoiding a targeted personal review by transitioning out of your position for several reasons: you have other more attractive opportunities (see Chap. 38); you no longer find the current position desirable (see Chap. 37); or you believe that the review is a means to unfairly dismiss you as chair. Some chairs simply find the thought of a targeted review (especially external) of their performance or behavior too threatening and prefer not to undergo the process. However, many individuals within and outside the institution will assume the apparent basis for a targeted review (e.g., poor performance, inappropriate behavior) is correct if you decide to resign rather than proceed with the review, so you should weigh a decision to avoid it very carefully.

Purpose of Department Reviews

"What Are the Expectations of a Department Review?"

Department reviews may be internal, external, or a combination of both and initiated for several reasons with different expectations. Most commonly, they are conducted towards the end of your current term to assess performance of both you and the department. Most institutions have a well-established process for conducting departmental reviews [2–4], and some professional organizations also have published templates for conducting reviews [5]. These reviews (especially external ones) are used to:

- Evaluate the department's performance under your leadership
- Assess gaps, opportunities, and strengths as a basis for strategic planning
- Establish goals and priorities
- Foster continuous improvement of programs
- Provide feedback to you and institutional leaders on performance improvement

In cases where you are eligible and desiring a subsequent term, the review also may provide specific recommendations about your reappointment. If you are not a candidate for renewal, the review usually will include issues and concerns facing the department with recommendations on the priorities needed for a new chair, which will be an important part of the subsequent search process. Occasionally a "targeted" department review may be initiated solely to address a specific operational or organizational question (e.g., should the department be merged with another; should the department change its structure; should space or finances be reallocated). Such reviews may or may not include a review of your performance and usually will only provide very specific recommendations regarding the issue being reviewed for you and the institution's leaders to consider.

Preparing for a Department Review

"How Do I Get Ready for a Review of My Department?"

Preparation for your department review will depend upon the type of review being conducted. Targeted department reviews that are focused on certain discrete areas of concern may be internal and only require gathering materials appropriate for that area, while comprehensive external reviews will require far more preparation. For comprehensive reviews, it is wise to conduct a departmental self-study prior to the review.

The self-study is a major effort that should be handled by several team leaders overseeing different aspects of the department including research, clinical service, education, outreach, and administrative functions (e.g., finance, communications, development). Anonymous surveys of department faculty, staff, trainees, and students often are conducted as a part of the self-study in order to evaluate their perspectives on the overall performance of the department and your effectiveness as the chair. Additional materials often include, but are not limited to:

- Listing of department faculty with their curricula vitae
- Organizational charts for the department and each division
- Maps of departmental space
- Financial statements
- Grant support
- Department strategic plan
- Program accreditations and certifications
- CME programs
- DEI efforts
- Philanthropic support

Although there is considerable variation from institution to institution, many department reviews utilize committees comprised of faculty from within the institution and several external to the institution, while others consist entirely of external reviewers. In order to maximize objectivity, there is usually no representation from the department on a review committee. Most information about the department is provided by the self-study, and additional information can always be requested from the department during the review.

As department chair, you may be asked to provide a letter outlining your evaluation of the department, its progress since the last review, issues that need to be addressed, and potential opportunities. You also may be asked to provide a list of potential external reviewers to serve on the committee, a list of referees to write letters of evaluation about your performance as chair, and a list of representative faculty members to be interviewed by the committee. In all of these situations you must ensure that any conflict of interest (real or perceived) in recommending committee members, reviewers, or interviewed faculty is fully disclosed.

Review "Etiquette"

"What Are the 'Do's and Don'ts' for Me in the Department Review Process?"

As department chair, you often will be the first and the last individual to be interviewed in the department and likely will be asked to present an overview of the department at the start of the review. If not requested previously, it also is advisable to have a written narrative assessment of the department, which should be included with the department self-study. At the interview itself you should be prepared to provide a finely tuned presentation that accurately describes the department's accomplishments during the period covered by the review. You should also include issues and concerns about the department, areas for improvement, potential opportunities, and future goals. You should be gracious and indicate your interest in learning the reviewers' assessment of your department and their recommendations. After the committee has obtained information from other interviews, it is not unusual for it to call back the chair to clarify issues raised during discussions.

If the department review is at the end of your term and you desire to be reappointed as chair, you should be straightforward during your closed session with the committee about your interest and priorities for the future. If you are stepping down as chair or leaving for another position, you should be candid in discussing the reasons, especially if they would be helpful to the department and your successor (e.g., the need for more resources).

Throughout the process you must resist any temptation to ask committee members about committee deliberations. The committee's discussions are strictly confidential, and any attempt to breach confidentiality can result in an invalidated review and even a negative review, for it may be viewed as attempted manipulation of the review committee.

Dealing with the Review Report

"How Should I React to the Review Report, Especially If It Is Not Entirely Positive?"

Most department reviews are conducted over 1–3 days on-site (or virtually) following prior review of submitted materials. At the conclusion of the site visit, the review committee normally prepares a preliminary draft report with recommendations regarding the department and your reappointment (if appropriate), which are discussed privately with institutional leaders. The information in this verbal report may be shared with you by leadership, or held back until receiving the review committee's final written report, which may differ a bit from their verbal report based on the feedback they receive from the leaders who engaged them.

If you consider the review to be less than favorable, you should not summarily reject it as flawed, especially if the review panel was duly constituted and charged. Instead, look at the report as a roadmap to improve the performance of you and your department. Before sharing it (redacted as appropriate) with the rest of the department and others, it is best to discuss the report's evaluation and recommendations with your institutional leadership and then your department leadership team, especially regarding follow-up plans.

You will need the support of your departmental and institutional leader(s) to develop a plan that will address committee recommendations. Failure to share the report in at least some form with your department will usually lead to rumors about a cover-up of weaknesses and problems. You should respond to the review in writing and discuss the department's plan and anticipated timeline to address suggested recommendations with your institutional leadership for their agreement and support.

Dealing with Program and Institution Reviews

"How Should I Handle Program, Accreditation, and Institution Reviews That Involve My Department?"

In addition to your departmental and personal reviews, you and your department may be involved in a variety of other reviews that involve your parent institutions, including medical school accreditation by the Liaison Committee on Medical Education (LCME), hospital accreditation by The Joint Commission (TJC), institutional animal use certification by the Association for Assessment and Accreditation of Laboratory Animal Care (AAALAC), and programmatic accreditations such as clinical laboratory certification by the College of American Pathologists (CAP), Comprehensive Cancer Center designation by the National Cancer Institute (NCI), Comprehensive Cardiac Center designation by the American Heart Association, and Trauma Center verification by the American College of Surgeons (ACS).

Each of these accreditation processes is highly organized, comprehensive, and complex, so that your involvement likely will be well directed by the appropriate institutional team involved in the process. While time-consuming, it is important as a good institutional team player for you and your department to be fully committed to participate as expected to help ensure positive outcomes. A lot is at stake for your institutions with these reviews, and any problems with your engagement would have significant negative consequences.

Similarly, you and your department will be engaged in accreditation reviews of your residency program by the ACGME and continuing education programs by the Accreditation Council for Continuing Medical Education (ACCME), among others. In addition to having the departmental directors of these programs taking the lead in handing these reviews, it is important for you to ensure full collaboration of faculty and staff in these review processes; a negative outcome would reflect poorly on you and the department and adversely impact your department's reputation and resident recruitment.

References

1. Buller JL. The essential department chair: a comprehensive desk reference. 2nd ed. Jossey-Basss; 2012. ISBN 978-1118123744.
2. Cornell University. Academic program review. https://irp.dpb.cornell.edu/academic-program-regulation/academic-program-review. Accessed 29 Mar 2023.
3. Princeton University. Guidelines for academic reviews. https://dof.princeton.edu/guidelines-academic-reviews/academic-review-process. Accessed 19 Oct 2022.
4. Stanford University. Departmental review guide. https://planning-humsci.stanford.edu/planning-processesdepartment-external-reviews/departmental-review-guide. Accessed 19 Oct 2022.
5. Collins J, Amis ES Jr, Beauchamp NJ Jr, Norbash AM, Meltzer CC. A guide to the external review of an academic radiology department. Acad Radiol. 2013;21:400–6. https://doi.org/10.1016/j.acra.2013.11.020.

Chapter 36
Achieving Work-Life Balance

Importance of Work-Life Balance

"How Can I Achieve a Successful Work-Life Balance?"

For many department chairs, more time is spent in a reactive rather than in a proactive mode. Chairs face unrelenting problems that require a response and easily can become controlled by their environment. Reactive chairs often have little time for their personal health and welfare, which also has a negative effect upon their loved ones and, in turn, exacerbates their own stress. Accordingly, they may become less productive, bitter, and burned out [1]. Moreover, burnout and loss of professional fulfillment in physician leaders have been shown to be significantly associated with their diminished effectiveness [2].

Successful chairs learn quickly that to survive the continuous demands of their job it is essential to have a good work-life balance, which requires careful and proactive time management. Juggling the priorities of your work is a challenge and includes the time demands of your institution(s), your department, and your own professional activities. As an institutional leader responsible for your department, you must make sure that your department is meeting the needs and expectations of its members as well as the institution. Sometimes, this will come at the expense of your own professional activities, which is a price paid by good leaders. However, balancing your overall work time commitment should not come at the expense of personal time, which is absolutely necessary to ensure the resilience and work-life satisfaction you need to be successful in your work as well as your personal life.

To manage your priorities effectively, you should schedule all your institutional, departmental, and professional work-related activities with an appropriate amount of unstructured work time each day to deal with unanticipated problems and emergencies, as well as to think creatively about your department and your personal scholarship. In addition, you should schedule an appropriate amount of

F. Sanfilippo et al., *Lead, Inspire, Thrive*,
https://doi.org/10.1007/978-3-031-41177-9_36

uninterrupted time for personal activities each day. Finding appropriate work-life balance does not just happen; you really have to work at it [3].

"As a Department Chair, Should I Even Consider Taking a Sabbatical Leave?"

As a department chair you may feel that it is inappropriate or selfish for you to take a sabbatical leave or, depending on institutional policy, a leave in lieu of sabbatical. The decision of whether or not to take a leave is dependent upon your individual circumstances. If you are a newly appointed chair (particularly from the outside), it may not be wise to leave your department while you are in the process of organizing it and aligning department priorities with those of the institution. However, after you have things under control and certainly by the time you progress to another term, you may feel confident enough to consider taking a sabbatical leave, particularly if you have built a strong team to lead the department in your absence. Remember that you are also a faculty member and probably under more stress than other faculty due to your leadership and administrative responsibilities. Thus, in many respects, you well deserve a sabbatical leave for your own career development and wellness (see Chap. 18).

Depending upon departmental and institutional specifics, sabbatical leaves may be for varying lengths of time, ranging from one or more "mini-sabbaticals" to a more traditional 6–12-month sabbatical leave. Although sabbaticals are usually taken externally, with instructions that you should be contacted only in dire emergencies, they sometimes are taken "in residence" (at one's own institution), in which case you may allow yourself to be contacted for urgent matters.

Some chairs may fear loss of control over their departments if they take a full sabbatical leave away from their institution and may have concern about the department languishing in their absence. If you harbor those fears, you may not have developed sufficient self-confidence in yourself and in your abilities to create a strong leadership team (see Chap. 33, section "Characteristics of Successful Leaders").

Finally, if circumstances do not allow you to take a sabbatical leave while serving as chair, you may wish to consider taking such a leave after you step down as chair, especially if you are returning to the faculty. In addition to allowing you to "re-tool" your research, clinical, and education skills, this may be a particularly efficacious way of allowing your successor as chair (interim or permanent) to run the department without feeling that their predecessor is watching them.

Time Management at Work

"What Are Strategies for Managing My Work Schedule?"

Starting with the day new chairs are announced, the number of their e-mails, texts, and phone calls increases dramatically, as does the number of meetings requested. From that point on, workload demands become substantially greater and rarely let up. To cope, most chairs start to overschedule appointments and increase multitasking, which can result in a diminished ability to focus and pay attention. In addition, the explosion of virtual meetings has been both a blessing and a curse with respect to time commitment and workload—good because it avoids nonproductive travel time to meetings (especially those which are off-site and distant), and bad because it results in many more meetings scheduled within the same timeframe. There also have been additional demands made on chairs who are women or members of underrepresented groups in order to enhance diversity on committees and projects (see Chap. 7).

Substantial advice is readily available from the literature, online, and from courses on how you can manage time at work. Perhaps the most important practice you should develop is having strict control of your calendar and schedule. This can be done by personally scheduling your own meetings, calls, events etc., which is extremely distracting, time-consuming, and generally not practical. A more effective approach is to have all scheduling handled by a trusted assistant (or assistants) who clearly knows your priorities and style, knows when to say no to a request, and knows when to bring you requests that are ambiguous.

Although allowing more than one assistant to access your appointment calendar directly can sometimes create problems in controlling your workload, it may be necessary depending on the magnitude and scope of your activities. As long as those with access to your calendar know your rules for scheduling, and work closely together, this can be an advantage rather than a problem.

You should also make sure that all parties know that scheduled times are considered pending until you personally approve them and, even then, are subject to last minute changes if necessary. A good practice at the end of your workday is to review for approval (or not) all new items that were scheduled during the day, and review your appointments for the following day with your assistant to determine if any changes are needed.

Handling Appointments

"How Can I Handle All the Appointments Requested?"

In handling meeting requests, you should first consider how long they need to be, especially if they are with your department's faculty, staff, students, and trainees. In most cases, you should limit such meetings to no more than 30 min, and the requester(s) should be asked at the time of scheduling to send you a brief agenda beforehand. This will allow you to prepare for the meeting and will save everyone time in discussing and resolving issues. This also will help you to determine whether the meeting is necessary, if others can handle the issue, and who else might be asked to participate.

If the meeting is not important enough for the requester(s) to send an agenda in a timely manner, you should cancel the meeting. This will help send the message that you take meetings seriously by preparing beforehand, and that they should too. That said, exceptions should be considered for students and trainees and of course for genuine emergencies.

If the meeting is with a faculty or staff member who has an intermediary or direct supervisor (e.g., division chef, vice chair, manager), be sure that they were involved in trying to resolve the issue before your meeting, and that the meeting is not an attempt to bypass their authority. The same should apply to students and trainees regarding their course director or training supervisor. Unless the meeting is about a confidential personal, performance, or grievance issue with their intermediary/superior, you should cancel the meeting until the requester has vetted the issue with them appropriately. This will help send the message that the leadership team in the department should be accessed appropriately, and that you do not want to bypass their involvement (see Chaps. 11, 20, 23, and 27).

"How Can I Use Meeting Time More Effectively?"

A very useful practice for all appointments is to add at least 10–15 min before and after each one to prepare properly, as well as to take notes afterward that include a brief summary and any specific follow-up plans. This is especially important when meeting with institutional leaders and when dealing with difficult or complex issues. Although adding extra time at both ends of meetings shortens the available time for appointments during the day, it will increase the value and effectiveness of meetings substantially and reduce your stress by not jumping from one appointment to the next being unprepared and having notes to remember what was discussed and needs to be done.

Although increasingly common, it is advisable not to plan anticipated work during virtual appointments. If the virtual activity consumes your attention, the anticipated work won't get done, and if you work during the virtual activity you may miss important items that warranted scheduling the virtual activity in the first place. Not paying attention during a virtual meeting is often recognized by others in attendance and can raise questions about how serious you are in meeting commitments. It can also be embarrassing to be called upon and not respond or have to say you were not paying attention.

Apart from appointments, be sure to schedule unstructured personal work time to deal with your "to-do" list and allow for unanticipated interruptions and unscheduled emergency meetings. As commonly advised, it is helpful to categorize your work as important/urgent, important/not urgent, not important/urgent, and routine, and keeping them in a work folder for easy access during your scheduled (and unscheduled) personal work time. Deciding what is urgent and what is important is often difficult because of so many competing priorities; a common mistake is to have urgent but less important items take precedence over the more important items simply because of the temptation to get them done sooner. It is interesting how often many urgent (but relatively unimportant) tasks can sit in a folder and become resolved on their own or simply disappear.

Enhancing Resilience

"How Can I Increase My Resilience to Stress?"

Resilience is the ability of an individual to respond to stress such that personal goals are accomplished at minimal physical and psychological cost. Resilient individuals not only recover rapidly after challenges but often grow stronger in the process [4]. One of the most common barriers to resilience is an imbalance between work and personal life [5]. You should make sure to have time for leisure activities in order to relieve stress and strengthen your resilience. Physical activity as well as cultural engagement (music, literature, art) may be particularly useful in this regard, along with the ability to perceive the positive things that occur in everyday professional life without taking them for granted [6]. Chairs and other leaders are often their own worst enemies, sacrificing themselves for their positions. You must realize that you cannot be effective in your position without taking care of yourself first.

Time for Family and Friends

"How Can I Ensure That My Work Schedule Does Not Preclude Time with Family and Friends?"

Finding time for your family and friends must be an explicit priority or it will become very limited from the demands of work. You should try to schedule family events, including vacations, well in advance and resist any encroachment from work-related activities. As everyone knows, but often forgets until too late, time with children and elderly parents is limited and soon gone forever, while work is always there.

Too many chairs and other leaders say late in their careers that their greatest regret was not spending more time with their spouses/partners, children as they were growing up, and parents who subsequently passed away. Very few will say they regretted not spending more time at work. You should get in the habit when pressed for time at work that risks your time with family of reminding folks that you believe in "Family First." Most will respect this attitude; those who don't may not share your values of family and friends and clearly don't understand the importance of work-life balance.

Personal Time

"How Can I Find Time Just to Relax and Have Fun?"

Unfortunately, chairs and other leaders often feel guilty for taking time away from work for their own recreational activities. The detrimental physical and mental effects of overwork on stress and sleep are well documented, as are the benefits of free time for personal reflection and social interactions. Making time for oneself is essential in order to stay refreshed, reduce stress, improve resilience, and avoid burnout. Limiting personal time to vacations is not enough. As noted above, time for hobbies, sports, physical exercise, fun with family and friends, personal appointments (including medical care), and simple rest and relaxation should be an essential part of your everyday life.

Extended personal time for vacations is also important for good work-life balance. Many find that at least two continuous weeks of true vacation are really needed to unwind from the stress and pressure of work and to truly become refreshed. The broad availability of remote access communication makes it much easier to vacation and still stay connected if needed for an emergency at work. This is beneficial if used in a very limited fashion for only the most urgent and essential functions. Unfortunately, if overused it can destroy the intended benefit of the time meant to be away from work and actually increase rather than reduce stress.

Rather than feeling guilty for taking personal time away from work, you should appreciate how it benefits your physical and mental health, strengthens your social connection with family and friends, and makes you a more effective role model and productive leader.

References

1. Shanafelt TD, Hasan O, Dyrbye LN, Sinsky C, Satele D, Sloan J, et al. Changes in burnout and satisfaction with work-life balance in physicians and the general US working population between 2011 and 2014. Mayo Clin Proc. 2015;90:1600–13. https://doi.org/10.1016/j.mayocp.2015.08.023.
2. Shanafelt TD, Makowski MS, Wang H, Bohman B, Leonard M, Harrington RA, et al. Association of burnout, professional fulfillment, and self-care practices of physician leaders with their independently rated leadership effectiveness. JAMA Netw Open. 2020;3:e207961. https://doi.org/10.1001/jamanetworkopen.2020.7961.
3. Editor. Balancing your life at work and home. J Oncol Pract. 2009;5:253–5. https://doi.org/10.1200/jop.091018.
4. Epstein RM, Krasner MS. Physician resilience: what it means, why it matters, and how to promote it. Acad Med. 2013;88:301–3. https://doi.org/10.1097/ACM.0b013e318280cff0.
5. Mahmoud NN, Rothenberger D. From burnout to well-being: a focus on resilience. Clin Colon Rectal Surg. 2019;32:415–23. https://doi.org/10.1055/s-0039-1692710.
6. Zwack J, Schweitzer J. If every fifth physician is affected by burnout, what about the other four? Resilience strategies of experienced physicians. Acad Med. 2013;88:382–9. https://doi.org/10.1097/ACM.0b013e318281696b.

Chapter 37
Career Transitioning

Knowing When It's Time

"How Do I Know When It Is Time to Transition?"

Modes of transitioning from department leadership include those that are planned proactively (e.g., taking another leadership position, stepping down from leadership roles, retirement) and those that are imposed and reactive (e.g., termination or non-renewal, personal and family issues). Ideally, proactive plans to transition are for positive reasons such as successful accomplishment of your goals or consideration of potentially attractive opportunities (see Chap. 38). However, in many instances proactive transition planning is initiated for other reasons including:

- You are no longer stimulated and satisfied by the position.
- You are spending most of your time on management rather than leadership.
- You do not feel appreciated or supported by your department or the institution.
- Your boss has been replaced with someone having different values and priorities.
- You do not have resources available for future progress and success of the department.
- You do not have the personal resources to be successful professionally.

Chairs and other leaders should consider transitioning while they have energy, ideas, and opportunities to work on something engaging either inside or outside of their field, especially while the department is still strong and on an upward trajectory [1]. If the desire to transition is due to burnout, consider first taking a leave of absence with intervention to reduce stress and enhance resilience, which may alleviate the problem [2]. Alternatively, you may wish to consider a sabbatical leave (see Chap. 36, section "Importance of Work-Life Balance").

F. Sanfilippo et al., *Lead, Inspire, Thrive*,
https://doi.org/10.1007/978-3-031-41177-9_37

"How Long Is Too Long to Serve as a Department Leader?"

A chair's cycle for implementing their vision and achieving expected goals is typically 7–10 years, although there are many exceptions. Regardless of the length of service, progress should be evident within the first 5 years, which is the minimum time a leader should plan to be committed to their role [3]. Leaving your position as chair too early can disrupt department progress and performance, as well as your reputation for not having completed what you started. However, remaining in the same leadership position for too long also may not be beneficial for you or the department.

Long-term service can result in your becoming addicted to the position and thinking of yourself more as representing the position than as a temporary steward of the department. Likewise, too much satisfaction with the status quo can set in with prolonged service, resulting in less innovation and greater resistance to change, which can lead to departmental members becoming more reluctant to bring issues forward, creating a vicious cycle of inertia.

Reciprocally, long-term leadership service can be beneficial by providing you more experience with departmental issues and opportunities, greater familiarity with department faculty/staff and institutional peers/leaders, as well as a better understanding of institutional policy and procedures, all of which can facilitate departmental initiatives. These benefits also can reduce some stress of the position and improve your work-life balance (see Chap. 36).

The best way to determine when to leave your leadership role is by having a high degree of self-awareness (see Chap. 33, section "Developing and Maintaining Self-Awareness"), which is tied to receiving ongoing candid feedback from colleagues and leaders in the department and institution (see Chap. 28) and getting advice from trusted mentors, friends, and family who know you well (see Chap. 34). Understanding the importance of feeling satisfaction as well as success with your work and confidence that your superiors are supporting as well as engaging you personally are subtle but important factors in knowing when it may be time to consider moving on.

Considering Options

"What Transition Opportunities Should I Consider?"

A common adage among chairs and other leaders after they leave a position is "There really is life after _____" (fill in the blank with your current leadership role). For successful individuals, the opportunities following their current leadership positions often are focused on other attractive leadership positions [4], which often present themselves unexpectedly (see Chap. 38).

If you are not retiring or moving to another leadership role, it is important to develop a transition plan early on that considers all options of potential interest [5], such as teaching, research, engaging in clinical work, writing, mentoring, becoming more active in professional organizations and boards, performing philanthropic work, or moving to another career entirely [1, 2]. Your relative interest in these and other career options will likely change over time, so it is advisable to update your transition (i.e., career) planning on a regular basis.

Imposed Termination

"How Best to Transition from an Imposed Termination?"

The most difficult transitions for leaders usually are those resulting from termination. These are high-stress situations that can have many different causes with many different outcomes depending on how they are handled. Most nonrenewals and terminations (except for cause) are handled carefully by those to whom you report, and they will often allow you to step down for "personal reasons" or "to pursue new opportunities" to minimize harm to both reputations. Ironically, some institutional leaders do not appreciate that terminating a chair whom they recruited can have a negative reflection on them and their institution for making a poor selection or not providing the appropriate support for the chair's success.

Likewise, how institutional leadership handles your termination will be viewed closely by those in and outside the institution and, if not done sensitively, can significantly damage their reputation. Therefore, unless termination is for cause, most institution leaders will try to help you make the transition as easy as possible. In these situations, it is wise to work prudently to negotiate the best transition possible. This should include detailed plans for the announcement and for recognition ("thank-you") events. Denigrating the individuals to whom you report (or your institution), even in private, will usually get back to them and be counter-productive in your negotiations or at some point in the future. And many who hear them will consider your disparaging remarks as a poor reflection on you.

Succession Planning

"When Should I Start My Succession Planning for My Department?"

The decision to leave your position before a permanent successor is named creates a difficult period for both you and the department because you no longer hold authority and an interim chair is not usually fully empowered. In addition, returning to the faculty is often awkward for both you and your successor (see Chap. 4) [3].

Succession planning allows institutional leaders to sustain and revitalize their organization by ensuring successful leadership transitions. Ideally, you should begin succession planning between 1 and 2 years after your initial appointment to help provide your institution with a contingency in case your service is unexpectedly cut short [6]. Identification of potential interim leaders in your department is an important part of such contingency succession planning.

Coping with Transition

"How Do I Deal with No Longer Being the Department Leader?"

If you step down from your leadership position and remain in the department, you may experience a sense of loss, exhilaration, or ambivalence. Your lack of authority and being out of the information loop may be difficult to accept, and you may be disappointed that your successor does not seek your advice. These feelings are normal, particularly if you have been in your leadership position for a long while. You can try to assuage them by focusing on how you might be of service to the department and your successor and becoming engaged without being intrusive or threatening to any departmental leaders. This might include volunteering to take on special projects that utilize your expertise (e.g., redesign of the department's website, revising curricula, launching new fellowship programs, working on an affiliation project).

Likewise, using your experience (and potentially some newfound time) may allow you to initiate projects such as writing books, creating elective courses in your discipline, and becoming more involved in mentoring faculty. Some professional organizations have sections for former department leaders to continue providing service to their organizations by sharing their experience and wisdom with other faculty and chairs in their discipline [7].

As noted above, before you step down from your leadership position, you should create a written plan for your activities and discuss it with family and friends as well as mentors and coaches. Think carefully about what your daily routine will be like and how you will divide the time previously spent in running the department on your own professional and personal pursuits.

References

1. Bailey DN, Buja LM, Gorstein F, Gotlieb A, Green R, Kane A, et al. Life after being a pathology department chair III; reflections on the "afterlife". Acad Pathol. 2019;6:2374289519846068. https://doi.org/10.1177/2374289519846068.
2. Bailey DN, Buja LM, Gotlieb AI, Powell DE, Sanfilippo F. Career transitions: reflections of former chairs and academic health leaders. Acad Pathol. 2022;9:100037. https://doi.org/10.1016/j.acpath.2022.100037.
3. Ness RB, Samet JM. How to be a department chair of epidemiology: a survival guide. Am J Epidemiol. 2010;172:747–51. https://doi.org/10.1093/aje/kwq268.
4. Bailey DN, Lipscomb MF, Gorstein F, Wilkinson D, Sanfilippo F. Life after being a pathology department chair: issues and opportunities. Acad Pathol. 2016;3:2374289516673651. https://doi.org/10.1177/2374289516673651.
5. Dodds DW, Cruz OS, Israel H. Attitudes toward retirement of ophthalmology department chairs. Ophthalmology. 2013;120:1502–5. https://doi.org/10.1016/j.ophtha.2012.12.023.
6. Rayburn W, Grigsby K, Brubaker L. The strategic value of succession planning for department chairs. Acad Med. 2016;91:465–8. https://doi.org/10.1097/ACM.0000000000000990.
7. Sanfilippo F, Markwood P, Bailey DN. Retaining the value of former department chairs: the association of pathology chairs experience. Acad Pathol. 2020;7:2374289520981685. https://doi.org/10.1177/2374289520981685.

Chapter 38
Changing Positions

Becoming a Candidate

"How Do I Become a Candidate for an Attractive Position Without Damaging My Current Department?"

You should first determine why you want to become a candidate for another position, even if it is another chair [1]. Is it the lure of the new position ("the pull") or are you becoming dissatisfied or bored with your current position ("the push")? These considerations are not unlike those encountered by candidates for their first leadership positions [2–4].

There are several approaches to being asked to become a candidate. An obvious way is to simply apply for an advertised position. Often a better strategy is to ask a trusted mentor, advisor, or colleague to nominate you for that position (see Chap. 34, section "Sponsors"). Sometimes, it is ideal to visit an institution as a guest (e.g., invited lecturer, speaker for a colleague's course) rather than (or before) officially applying to see if the position feels like a good fit. In some instances, even if a position is not posted, writing a letter indicating your interest in a leadership position at another institution may serve to get you on the radar screen of that institution so that when an appropriate opportunity becomes available you may be asked to apply. Finally, maintaining both formal and informal interactions with search firm recruiters can be helpful as they are incentivized to cultivate confidential lists of candidates for multiple leadership opportunities.

If you are asked to become a candidate for a position and might be interested, you should indicate your willingness to explore the opportunity at the other institution, even if you are satisfied with your current position. This will give you the opportunity to learn more about another institution and the way they do things, as well as to develop new colleagues and potential collaborations. If you are not

F. Sanfilippo et al., *Lead, Inspire, Thrive*, https://doi.org/10.1007/978-3-031-41177-9_38

interested, you should explicitly say so and offer a cogent reason (e.g., you are satisfied where you are, why the new position is not a good fit for you).

If, after an initial interview, you decide to become a formal candidate, it is wise to let those to whom you report know that you are exploring a new position. Academic leadership is a fairly small group, and word travels quickly. It is better to tell your institutional leaders about becoming a candidate than if they hear it from another source and potentially misinterpret your reason for not telling them. Being transparent about considering other positions can actually enhance your relationship with institutional leaders, especially if you ask for their advice. Reciprocally, being silent or deceptive may damage your relationship with them, which can be very detrimental if you stay.

Interviews and Visits

"How Do I Handle Interviews and Visits for Another Position While I'm Still Running My Department?"

First-round (screening) interviews are relatively simple and may, in fact, be conducted virtually. Even when in person, first interviews usually occupy only 1 day. This is a relatively small time commitment and should not interfere with running your department. The screening interview allows both parties (you and the other institution) to evaluate the relative degree of interest and potential fit on both sides and whether to proceed. If you are invited for a formal on-site visit, you may wish to inform those to whom you report, as mentioned above. In so doing, you should indicate that you simply are exploring an interesting opportunity but are far from making any decisions.

For institutions with public search processes, it is advisable to let your leadership and department know you are looking even for a first screening visit, and that you will keep them apprised if it becomes more likely. Before your first visit, do your homework. Research the background of everyone with whom you will interview, know their interests and their accomplishments, and where they sit in the administrative hierarchy. Study the history of the institution and its departments. Be sure you are ready to indicate why you may be interested in the new position, especially relative to your current one.

If a second visit is scheduled, you should let your institutional leadership and your department know immediately, because second visits usually signal serious interest in the position, and they will undoubtedly hear about it from other sources.

Evaluating the Opportunity

"How Do I Determine If Taking a New Position Is the Right Change to Make?"

In evaluating a new leadership opportunity, listen to both your head and your heart. Carefully consider some key issues:

- The professional advantages and disadvantages of the new position.
- The impact on your career and that of your colleagues, students, and trainees.
- Tangible factors (e.g., compensation, retirement benefits, relocation issues).
- The effects on your family and friends.

If your head and your heart are not in alignment, you should carefully assess why there is a disparity. In many cases it is worth making a very objective and weighted comparison of all the factors that are of importance to get an "objective" assessment. Often your heart will put too much weight on some factors and not enough on others, so it is important to include objective comparisons of even "subjective" factors in your assessment.

One of the most important factors to consider in looking at a new position is how well you will fit into the culture of that organization, especially if you are being asked to drive significant changes there (see Chap. 6). It also is critical to be sure that the roles and responsibilities you are being offered are aligned with the authority being provided. Finally, be sure that you can succinctly describe why you are interested in the position and what value you can bring to it and to the institution. Above all, be transparent so the recruiting institution's leaders can assess your interest accurately and how well you would fit into the role being filled. Avoid using your candidacy for another position as leverage to improve your circumstances at your own institution. Even the perception of doing so can be damaging for your reputation, your current position, and the interest of the recruiting institution.

Closing the Deal

"How Should I Finalize the Agreement for My New Position?"

When finalizing the terms of a new position, be thoughtful in negotiations with your future boss(es) (see Chap. 10). Utilizing intermediaries in the negotiation may be helpful and can often be arranged via the search firm if one was used. Negotiations should be focused on what will enable you to achieve the new institution's articulated goals. Be mindful of resources and indicate that you will ask only for what is essential to accomplish the goals and expectations set by the new institution. Remember that recruitment packages are not all about space, resources, and money; the autonomy and influence granted to you and the unit you will lead are also important factors. Keep the agreement for your own personal and professional resources separate from those needed for your leadership position. Bring lessons learned from your prior leadership experience to the table in these negotiations.

Leaving Gracefully

"How Do I Make the Right Exit from My Current Position to Another One?"

How you exit from your current position depends on why you are leaving. If you have been successful as a chair, this should be relatively easy. You should create a realistic timetable for leaving so that your current institution can implement the succession plan that you (hopefully) already have helped develop (see Chap. 37, section "Succession Planning"). If no succession plan is in place, your transition timetable might be prolonged to assure the stability of the department you are leaving. Providing recommendations for an interim chair is often appreciated [5].

Ideally, your transition timetable should be acceptable to both your current institution and your new one. If that is not possible, you should try to accommodate the wishes of your new institution since that will be your new home. If you are leaving your current institution because of modest (or lack of) success, you should be transparent about it and avoid disparaging the institution.

Whenever possible, indicate the benefits of your departure for the department and institution. Always leave on positive terms and be sure that you clear up any lingering problems as best you can before you leave your current department. Just as you don't want to deal with festering problems when you arrive in your new position, don't leave them for your successor.

Finally, in accepting another position, it is important to know when public disclosure of your appointment will be made. It is also important that your home institution knows before the information leaks out and that notices are appropriately staged to inform your old and new departments, old and new institutions, donors and key community leaders, and then the public.

Expect Surprises

"Did I Make the Right Decision in Changing Positions?

Not infrequently, after changing positions, you may wonder whether your decision to leave was correct, not unlike when you assumed your current role as chair. This may have several causes: the position was not described in sufficient detail and is not what you thought it would be; you did not do your homework in researching the position and find unanticipated problems after you arrive; the organizational culture and fit are not right for you; the onboarding process was deficient; recruitment promises are not being honored; or circumstances in your personal life have changed.

Although these or other factors may tempt you to leave your new position, you should resist the thought. Many issues resolve themselves over time. You must appreciate the fact that both your new position and the environment will be quite different than your former one and often will be more complex if you are moving to a more senior leadership role. It often just takes time to settle into the job and to learn to navigate in your new environment. If feelings of dissatisfaction persist after a year, you should have a serious talk with institutional leadership and consider your options. Leaving within a year or two after accepting a new position may be damaging to your reputation and to that of the institution.

References

1. Buller JL. The essential department chair: a comprehensive desk reference. 2nd ed. Jossey-Bass; 2012. ISBN 978-1118123744.
2. Bailey DN, Lipscomb MF, Gorstein F, Wilkinson D, Sanfilippo F. Life after being a pathology department chair: issues and opportunities. Acad Pathol. 2016;3:2374289516673651. https://doi.org/10.1177/2374289516673651.
3. Bailey DN, Lipscomb MF, Gorstein F, Wilkinson D, Sanfilippo F. Life after being a pathology department chair II: lessons learned. Acad Pathol. 2017;4:2374289517733734. https://doi.org/10.1177/2374289517733734.
4. Bailey DN, Buja LM, Gotlieb AI, Powell DE, Sanfilippo F. Career transitions: reflections of former chairs and academic health leaders. Acad Pathol. 2022;9:100037. https://doi.org/10.1016/j.acpath.2022.100037.
5. Fennah P, Steinberg B, Watkins MD. How to quit when you lead a team. Harv Bus Rev. 2022. https://hbr.org/2022/01/how-to-quit-when-you-lead-a-team. Accessed 29 Mar 2023.

Final Thoughts

As is often said, leadership is a journey, not a destination. And today, more than ever, the journey of a department chair can be demanding with frustrating road-blocks, unanticipated accidents, and grueling detours. At the same time, chairs have the special opportunity to advance inspiring missions of research, education, health care, and public service, benefit their organizations and fields of expertise, and support the aspirations and career development of others.

Medical school department chairs are called on to be inspirational leaders in the rapidly changing world of academic medicine. Guiding complex programs and expert faculty and staff requires a broad array of talents, including superlative "EQ" (Emotional Quotient) and interpersonal skills; sophisticated understanding of health care delivery and reimbursement; familiarity with new research approaches; enthusiasm for educating a diverse cadre of trainees; and commitment to academic medicine's unique social mission. Not only must chairs lead effectively in the current environment, but they also must position their department for success in quickly evolving and often unpredictable scenarios. By embracing a "future-oriented" perspective, chairs can inspire others and leave a powerful legacy.

As leaders we learn a lot over time. The more experience we have, the more we understand how much more we need to know. In the final analysis, a critical measure of a leader's accomplishment is their feeling of personal satisfaction. If this book helps chairs and other leaders find greater satisfaction in their roles, and helps them to lead, inspire, and thrive, then it has achieved its purpose.

Appendix A: Other Works Offering Advice for Academic Department Chairs

Allard C. The essentials for new department chairs. John Wiley & Sons; 2011. ISBN 978-1118196731.

Benisimon EM. The department chair's role in developing new faculty into teachers and scholars. Jossey-Bass; 2000. ISBN 978-1882982339.

Biebuyck JF. The successful medical school department chair, module 1: search, selection, appointment, transition. Association of American Medical Colleges; 2003. https://store.aamc.org/aamc-successful-medical-school-department-chair-series-the-complete-set-of-leading-recruiting-and-thriving-print.html.

Biebuyck JF. The successful medical school department chair, module 2: characteristics, responsibilities, expectations, skill sets. Association of American Medical Colleges; 2003. https://store.aamc.org/aamc-successful-medical-school-department-chair-series-the-complete-set-of-leading-recruiting-and-thriving-print.html.

Biebuyck JF. The successful medical school department chair, module 3: performance, evaluation, rewards, renewal. Association of American Medical Colleges; 2003. https://store.aamc.org/aamc-successful-medical-school-department-chair-series-the-complete-set-of-leading-recruiting-and-thriving-print.html.

Buller JL. The essential department chair: a comprehensive desk reference. 2nd ed. Jossey-Bass; 2012. ISBN 978-1118123744.

Buller JL, Cipriano RE. A toolkit for department chairs. Rowman and Littlefield; 2015. ISBN 978-1475814194. The Chronicle of Higher Education: A toolbox for department chairs. https://store.chronicle.com/collections/faculty-tag/products/a-toolbox-for-department-chairs (2022). Accessed September 1, 2023.

Chu D. The department chair primer: leading and managing academic departments. Wiley & Sons; 2008. ISBN 978-1882982936.

Chu D. The department chair primer: what chairs need to know and do to make a difference. 2nd ed. Jossey-Bass; 2012. ISBN 978-1118077443.

Chu D. The department chair field manual: a primer for academic leadership. (Independently Published); 2021. ISBN 979-8616773685.

Crookston RK. Working with problem faculty: a six-step guide for department chairs. Jossey-Bass; 2012. ISBN 978-1118242384.

Dettmar K. How to chair a department: higher ed. leadership essentials. Johns Hopkins University Press; 2022. ISBN 978-1421445236.

Gmelch WH, Miskin VD. Chairing an academic department. Atwood Publishing; 2004. ISBN 978-1891859526.

Grigsby RK, Mallon WT. Thriving: new perspectives and approaches for personal and organizational success. Association of American Medical Colleges; 2020. ISBN 978-1577541820.

Hansen CK. Time management for department chairs. Jossey-Bass; 2011. ISBN 978-0470769010.

Hecht, Irene WE, Higgerson ML, Gmelch WH, Tucker A. The department chair as academic leader. Rowman and Littlefield; 1998. ISBN: 978-1573561347.

Hey JAK. The balancing acts of academic leadership: a guide for department chairs and deans. Rowman and Littlefield; 2021. ISBN 978-1475855005.

Higgerson ML. Communication skills for department chairs. Jossey-Bass; 1996. ISBN 978-1882982134.

Jochum CJ. The department chair: a practical guide to effective leadership. Rowman and Littlefield; 2021. ISBN 978-1475862522.

Leaming DR. Academic leadership: a practical guide to chairing the department. Anker Publishing; 1998. ISBN 978-1933371177.

Leaming DR. Managing people: a guide for department chairs and deans. Jossey-Bass; 2003. ISBN 978-1882982530.

Lees ND. Chairing academic department: traditional and emerging expectations. Anker Publishing; 2002. ISBN 978-1933371030.

Lucas AE. Strengthening departmental leadership: a team-building guide for chairs in colleges and universities. Wiley & Sons; 1994. ISBN 978-0787900120.

Mallon WT, Grigsby RK. Leading: top skills, attributes, and behaviors critical for success. Association of American Medical Colleges; 2016. ISBN: 9781577541516.

Mallon WT, Grigsby RK. Recruiting: proven search and hiring practices for the best talent. Association of American Medical Colleges; 2017. ISBN: 978-157741684.

Sheff RA, Marder RJ. Department chair essentials handbook. Hcpro; 2012. ISBN 978-1601469465.

The Chronicle of Higher Education: A toolbox for department chairs. 2022. https://store.chronicle.com/collections/faculty-tag/products/a-toolbox-for-department-chairs. Accessed 18 Mar 2023.

Tucker A. Chairing the academic department: leadership among peers. Oryx Press; 1992. ISBN 978-0897748261.

Wheeler DW, Seagren AT, Becker LW, Kinley, E, Robson KT, Minek D. The academic chair's handbook. 2nd ed. Jossey-Bass; 2008. ISBN: 978-0470197653.

Wheeler DW, Creswell JW, Seagren AT. The department chair: new roles, responsibilities and challenges. Jossey-Bass; 1993. ISBN 13: 9781878380227.

Appendix B: References for General Reading

Barney J. Gaining and sustaining competitive advantage. 4th ed. Prentice Hall; 2010. ISBN 978-0136120926.

Chun E, Evans A. The department chair as transformative diversity leader: building inclusive learning environments in higher education. Stylus Publishing; 2015. ISBN 978-1620362389.

Conley A, Shaker G. Fundraising principles for Faculty and Academic Leaders. Palgrave Macmillan; 2021. ISBN 978-3030664282.

Dever C, Justice G: Leading from the middle: insight and advice for department chairs. The Chronicle of Higher Education. https://connect.chronicle.com/rs/931-EKA-218/images/LeadingFromtheMiddle.pdf?aliId=eyJpIjoid3RJTkpIQXBVNk5XbFRmZiIsInQiOiJHWHhZTjZJV1JcL0h3NDFOZUUd0MmJoQT09In0%253D. Accessed September 1, 2023.

Fisher R, Ury WL, Patton B. Getting to yes: negotiating agreement without giving in. Penguin Press; 2011. ISBN 978-0143118756.

Gasman M. Doing the right thing: how to undo systemic racism in faculty hiring. Princeton University Press; 2022. ISBN 978- 0691193076.

Heskett JL, Sasser WE, Schlesinger LA. What great service leaders know and do: creating breakthroughs in service firms. Berrett-Koehler Publishers; 2015. ISBN 978-1626565845.

Kotter JP. Leading change. Harvard Business Review Press; 2012. ISBN 978-1422186435.

Lees ND. Considerations for successfully "managing up." Acad Leader. 2014;30:1–6. https://www.academic-leader.com/topics/leadership/considerations_for_successfully_managing_up/.

Rucci AJ, Kirn SP, Quinn PE. The employee-customer-profit chain at Sears. Harv Bus Rev. 1998;76:82–97.

Souba WW, Notestine M, Way D, Yu L, Sedmak D. Do deans and teaching hospital CEOs agree on what it takes to be a successful clinical department chair? Acad Med. 2011;86:974–81. https://doi.org/10.1097/ACM.0b013e31822223b2.

Weaver LD, Ely K, Dickson L, DelAntonio J. The changing role of the department chair in the shifting landscape of higher education. Int J Higher Educ. 2019;8:175–88. https://doi.org/10.5430/ijhe.v8n4p175.

Appendix C: Glossary of Terms Used

Academic Freedom Academic freedom is the right of faculty to express their ideas and opinions without censorship, threat to their tenure or appointment, or institutional retaliation, but with limits on imposing their views on students, and requiring compliance with policies and laws against harassing, threatening, intimidating, or ridiculing others.

Academic Health Center (AHC) An academic health center encompasses all the health-related components of a university, including the health professions schools, patient care operations, and research enterprise (AAHC). Thus, the AHC might include one or more teaching hospitals and clinics, other affiliated hospitals and clinics, a medical school, and health professions schools (pharmacy, nursing, public health, dentistry, others). AHCs in the United States have a wide range of organizational governance and financing structures.

Academic Medical Center (AMC) Academic medical centers are organizations that vary in organization, ownership, governance, and operational models, and "range from stand-alone medical schools and independent teaching hospitals to university-based institutions that integrate multiple education, clinical and research sites." Commonly, the term AMC is used to refer to a tertiary care hospital and clinic system that is organizationally and administratively integrated with a medical school. In this book, we use the combined term AHC/AMC to include both types of organizations.

Career Development Career development is the process by which one advances through the stages of one's job and employment. It reflects the support that the organization provides to professional growth, including progressive advancement within the organization or transitions to new roles. This support can include coaching, mentoring, sponsorship, skills development, networking, wellness programs, and more.

© The Editor(s) (if applicable) and The Author(s), under exclusive license to
Springer Nature Switzerland AG 2023
F. Sanfilippo et al., *Lead, Inspire, Thrive*,
https://doi.org/10.1007/978-3-031-41177-9

Career Ladder Career ladders are delineated steps that outline the progression of jobs and roles in an organization, ranked in order of anticipated attainment based on training and scope of responsibility, and thus generally resulting in increasing compensation.

Center A center is a non-degree granting, often multidisciplinary, unit that has a specific mission (research, education, clinical) and that has faculty and other resources gathered from multiple departments and divisions. It may be physical or virtual.

Chair Package The chair package is the commitment of resources (e.g., salary, personnel, space, budgetary support, etc.) from the hiring authority that are made available to the new head of a department in order to meet the expectations of his or her new role. This includes resources both for the leader as an individual and for the department as a whole.

Chief Executive Officer The chief executive officer is the individual responsible for overseeing the administration of a large organization (e.g., hospital or AHC/AMC).

Clinical Enterprise The clinical enterprise consists of the parts of the AHC and AMC devoted to patient care delivery and health maintenance, including owned or affiliated hospitals, clinics, pharmacies, long-term care facilities, rehabilitation centers, faculty practices, etc., and the associated personnel, budgets, and other resources available to deliver that care.

Collaboration Collaboration is the act(s) of working jointly with others or together in a mutually agreed upon endeavor. Collaboration may occur between individuals or organizations.

Collegiality Collegiality is successful cooperative interaction among colleagues, especially when the group of colleagues takes collective responsibility for their work together, and when this work results in productive interpersonal exchanges, personal satisfaction, and effective outcomes.

Cultural Competence Cultural competence is the body of knowledge, interpersonal skills, behaviors, attitudes, and policies that enable health professionals to value and respect, as well as to understand, diverse cultures and their members. Culturally competent educators, researchers, and clinicians are able to use these understandings and skills to more effectively teach students, perform investigations, and treat patients from all communities in the way most appropriate for those they serve.

Department In academic medicine, a department is the organizational unit of a medical school devoted to a particular discipline. Departments generally group the faculty for purposes of hiring, promotion, and finances. In most cases, medical school departments include those devoted to the basic sciences (e.g., biochemistry, anatomy, etc.) and those aligned with clinical specialties (e.g., surgery, medicine, pediatrics, etc.). In some cases, departments may be formed to group faculty by roles such as education departments or research departments.

Development Development is the entire process of developing donors, performing fundraising, and maintaining stewardship of the donor.

Diversity, Equity, and Inclusion (DEI) Diversity, equity, and inclusion is a conceptual framework that seeks to promote the fair treatment and full participation of all people, especially in the workplace, including populations who have historically been excluded and been subject to discrimination and bias, resulting in their under-representation and lack of access to opportunities, because of their gender, race/ethnicity, sexual orientation, socioeconomic status, disability, or other aspects of their background, identity, or life experiences. Diversity is the presence of individuals, practices, and beliefs from different backgrounds, perspectives, and life experiences. Equity is the outcome of ensuring that policies, practices, and behaviors are fair and non-biased, and providing everyone the opportunity to achieve their maximal potential. Inclusion is the practice of making all individuals feel a sense of belonging and a belief that they are valued and respected.

Division Some medical school departments may have multiple divisions or sections, often related to subspecialty disciplines (e.g., cardiology, infectious disease, pediatric surgery, etc.).

Emeritus Faculty Emeritus faculty are individuals who have retired in good standing from an academic institution. Procedures for granting this title may vary from institution to institution with respect to required years of service, academic series, and position at the time of retirement.

Faculty Practice Plan Faculty practice plans are entities that provide services that support the professional practices of medical school clinicians, often including billing, collections, payor contracts, and revenue distribution. Plan structures vary considerably in governance, scope of authority, and relationship to the other parts of the academic health center.

Health Professions Schools Health professions schools are all the schools that are dedicated to educating future health professionals and may include medicine, osteopathy, pharmacy, dentistry, public health, nursing, veterinary medicine, "allied" professions, and others.

Inspire To inspire is to fill others with the desire to feel, believe, or do something, especially things that will fulfill them and allow them personal satisfaction and career success.

Institute　An institute is an organization, often multidisciplinary, whose focus usually is research. It typically has faculty from several different departments and a physical structure.

Institutional Leaders　For medical school department chairs, institutional leaders with whom they interact may include deans of the medical school, presidents or other university leaders, and/or hospital administrators, among others. Chairs most often report directly to the medical school dean, but may also report to others such as the hospital CEO in matrix organizations.

Lead　To lead is to guide another person by showing them the way and providing the resources that they need to attain the goal.

Medical School　Medical schools are organizations dedicated to educating and training the next generation of health leaders. They often have a four-part mission of education, clinical care, research, and public service. Schools in the United States have many different structures—they may be public or private, and are often part of a university but may be free-standing or created by a health system.

Ombudsperson　An ombudsperson is an individual who confidentially and impartially investigates, reports on, and helps to settle complaints, often through recommendations and/or remediation.

Organizational Culture　Organizational culture is the collection of values, expectations, and practices that guide, influence, and inform the actions of all the group's members.

Parent Institution　An organization that has governance and/or financial oversight responsibility over the referent organization. For medical school departments, parent institutions are usually universities, but may also include hospitals/health systems and for-profit investors.

Physician Self-Care　Physician self-care is the collection of strategies available to individual physicians to take better care of themselves. Such strategies can result in improved personal satisfaction, less burnout, and ultimately better ability to perform in their job.

Private University　A private university is an academic institution whose core (non-extramural) funding is predominately nonpublic. Private and public institutions are often held to different standards with respect to transparency and disclosure of items including salaries.

Public University　A public university is an academic institution whose core (non-extramural) funding is predominately nonprivate, usually from governmental (especially state) funding sources. Private and public institutions are often held to different standards with respect to transparency and disclosure of items including salaries.

Sabbatical Leave A sabbatical leave is a period of time for an employee to change workplaces in order to learn new skills, advance their career development, and refresh themselves professionally. Often the leave is at least partially (and occasionally fully) compensated.

Strategic Planning Strategic planning is the process by which the organization's members articulate their vision and mission and then identify and prioritize the strategies, tactics, and timelines (usually over 3 to 5 years) for advancing the mission. Strategic plans often include definition of metrics that will be used to assess progress, effectiveness, and impact.

Tenure Tenure is indefinite appointment (security of employment) that can be terminated only for cause or under extraordinary circumstances such as financial exigency. In academic institutions it is granted to eligible faculty after review of their achievements and accomplishments over a defined period of time. However, it is not necessarily a commitment of compensation level.

Thrive To thrive is to flourish and grow vigorously, both personally and professionally, allowing one to make important contributions, increase in stature, achieve impact, and be resilient, all while experiencing personal fulfillment. Thriving is an emotional, psychological, and behavioral state which positions one to effectively overcome challenges and take advantage of opportunities.

Trainee A trainee is an individual who is learning new skills to advance their career after receiving their degree. In AHCs/AMCs, these include house staff (medical interns and residents), fellows, and postdoctoral scholars among others.

Volunteer Faculty Volunteer faculty are individuals from other institutions who provide services (usually education or training) without compensation because they support the mission. At some institutions, they may be granted an academic title (e.g., adjunct or volunteer clinical professor). Occasionally they may generate clinical revenue, which could be paid to them through a staff contract instead of a faculty salary line.

Wellness Program A wellness program is a set of practices and offerings that serve to ensure that constituents thrive, especially in learning and/or work environments, and achieve personal comfort, satisfaction, and success.

Work-Life Balance Work-life balance is the state in which individuals achieve their desired equilibrium between the demands and satisfactions of their career and the demands and satisfactions of their personal life.

Appendix D: Chapter Summaries

Chapter 1: Introduction

- New and experienced medical school department chairs have many questions as they navigate the challenges and opportunities unique to their schools and associated AHC/AMCs.
- Medical school department chairs in clinical departments are distinct by having a healthcare enterprise mission in addition to education, research, and public service.
- Medical school department leadership requires complex alignment of priorities and resources across missions and organizations.
- Medical school departments are usually larger than departments in other parts of the university.
- Medical school department chairs are often recruited from the outside and typically serve longer terms than other university department chairs.
- Medical school department chairs often have more opportunities to garner resources through their clinical mission and associated development activities

Chapter 2: Setting Initial Goals

Starting Out

- Understand the organizational model of your medical school, and your scope of authority in the health systems that are used for your department's clinical service and training activities.
- Confirm that your authority as chair is consistent with the responsibilities designated and agreed on.

- Set your goals for the first 100 days in order to lay the foundation for your leadership.
- Base your goals on the expectations set by you, your institution, and your department.
- Make your goals specific, easily articulated, attainable, measurable, realistic, relevant, and time-based.
- Ensure that your goals reflect the charge you are given at recruitment and hiring.
- Involve your faculty and staff from the outset because their acceptance of the goals is essential.
- Determine what changes need to be made with your leadership team to achieve goals.
- Make sure reasons for changes are understood by all stakeholders.
- Track your goals regularly.
- Evaluate the resources provided in your recruitment in regard to expectations and goals.
- Keep resources provided for your personal and professional use separate from those for the department.
- Place department needs before your own needs.

Your Initial Message

- Understand that your initial message will lay the foundation and set the tone for your relationship with members of your department and institution.
- Ensure that your initial message lays out the goals, vision, and strategy for your department with the processes for achieving them.
- Include descriptions of your intended departmental organizational structure, processes for strategic planning and communication, and your management style.
- Indicate what is expected of you and the department.
- Be clear that your primary goal is the success of the department rather than individual gain.

Getting the Faculty and Staff Involved

- Involve faculty and staff in development of initial goals; engage them in a SWOT analysis.
- Consider using offsite retreats in developing goals and direction.

Getting External Help in Setting Goals

- Get advice and assistance from peer leaders (including new and established department leaders), consultants, and your professional societies for establishing initial goals.
- Evaluate your leadership skills and acquire/improve any that you feel are inadequate.

Chapter 3: Expectations

Measuring Your Success

- Meet with the individual(s) to whom you report and get written criteria for the measures of success that are expected for the department and you personally.
- Ensure that you receive annual appraisals with a list of objectives and benchmarks.
- Realize that your department will measure success by their accomplishments as a whole and not by your personal and professional achievements.
- Determine the measures of success that are of personal value and satisfaction.

Serving as an Interim Chair

- Understand that service as an interim chair may be useful if you are interested in becoming a future leader or if you want to make changes in the department without becoming the permanent chair.
- Determine the role expected (caretaker, manager, leader) and how you would deal with being a candidate for permanent chair or returning to the faculty.
- Evaluate your willingness to put your academic productivity at risk.

"Internal" Versus "External" Recruitment

- Appreciate that internal candidates have the potential benefits of better knowledge of the department and institution, and usually can begin sooner.
- Realize that internal candidates have the potential risks of preconceived biases and being perceived as receiving fewer resources.
- Understand that if you were an internal candidate you may be viewed as easier to manipulate.
- Realize that external chairs may have fresher, more objective ideas, but require more resources for relocation.

Prior Leadership Experience

- Understand that a risk of prior service as chair is having preconceived ways of addressing issues and opportunities in the new position.
- Realize that a benefit of prior service as chair is having more experience in handling issues and opportunities.

Surprises

- Appreciate that, regardless of whether you were an internal or external candidate, some unexpected issues and opportunities, as well as good and bad surprises, will occur.
- Realize that most new chairs wonder at some point if they made the correct decision in accepting the role.
- Remain resilient and do not let surprises overwhelm you.

Chapter 4: Dealing with Your Predecessor

Developing a Relationship

- Consider extending your previous relationship with the prior chair as a colleague or past member of their department, regardless of their success as former leader.
- Show respect and consideration to your predecessor; your behavior will be watched by many within and outside the department.
- Clearly delineate how you would like to communicate with your predecessor.
- Consider giving a well-defined title to your predecessor so that they understand their role and its boundaries.

Advice and Assistance

- Develop an understanding about when you will seek advice from your predecessor and when they should offer advice.
- Be careful not to imply that your predecessor is still running the department or that they have decision rights on issues or veto power over your decisions.

Dealing with Interference

- Treat interference by your predecessor as a special case of dealing with difficult faculty.
- Be careful how you deal with problems with your predecessor because there is substantial risk to both of your reputations and relationships.
- Remember that former chairs likely will have relationships with many internal and external stakeholders who they may engage to help pressure you.
- Handle requests for inappropriate support and resources with the same due consideration as with other faculty.
- Honor previous institutional commitments to your predecessor.
- Try to win over skeptical predecessors by gaining the confidence of your department and by successfully achieving goals and expectations.

Chapter 5: Communication

Enhancing Your Communication Skills

- Realize that communicating as a leader to stakeholders is different than as a professional to students and colleagues.
- Get an assessment of your speaking and writing skills and advice on how to improve your effectiveness from experts, including your institutional communications staff.
- Know your audience; communicate to their expectations, demographics, and knowledge level.
- Determine which communications tools and methods are best for you to use depending on urgency, complexity, the audience, and the need for documentation or confidentiality.
- Use e-mail as is a reliable, rapid, and efficient method of communication, and follow-up as necessary if an expected response is not received within an appropriate time frame.
- Use handwritten or typed/signed letters to convey personal gratitude and recognition.
- Appreciate that body language can play an important part of communication but can be misleading.

Transparency and Establishing Trust

- Remember that transparency, authenticity, and honesty are at the heart of good communication.
- Plan departmental meetings with an "open forum" and presentations from different sections.
- Solicit input, feedback, and advice from faculty, staff, and institutional leadership.
- Respond in a timely manner to communications, including e-mail, even if the response is a simple "thank you."
- Recognize achievements and awards by personal e-mail or notes along with appropriate announcements.
- Address malicious rumors and gossip by correcting inaccuracies, and avoiding broad responses.
- Understand the guarantees and limits of free speech and tradition of academic freedom, and address offensive speech with education and counseling.
- Communicate your department's mission, values, and expectations throughout the institution.

Accommodating Institutional Priorities and Reforms

- Explain the rationale and potential benefits of institutional priorities and changes to your department.

- Avoid disagreements and conflict with your institution's leaders over their decisions and priorities.
- Document unique contributions your department can make to facilitate proposed changes, especially in collaboration with other units.
- Determine the institutional and departmental impact and opportunity costs of changes in institutional policies and priorities.
- Invite your institution's leadership for a department meeting to discuss the rationale and potential impact of controversial changes.

Chapter 6: Organizational Culture

Understanding Culture Types and Styles

- Understand that departmental culture represents the norms and expectations of faculty, staff, trainee, and student behavior.
- Appreciate that culture is strongly related to values and can enhance or disrupt strategic plans and priorities.
- Recognize the different cultures that may be in different sections of your department.
- Know that organizational culture is tied to expectations, values, and behavior of the leader.
- Realize that culture may be affected by the type of organization and geopolitical influences.
- Learn about the general types of culture (passive, aggressive, and constructive) and the specific behavioral styles associated with each.

Evaluating Your Organizational Culture(s)

- Examine internal and external manifestations of culture through interactions with your faculty, staff, and students/trainees, and from stakeholders outside the department.
- Assess the level of faculty, staff, trainee, and student satisfaction with the current behavioral norms and expectations of your department.
- Determine the level of institutional satisfaction with your department's culture.
- Consider making a detailed evaluation of your department's culture using objective assessment tools.

Driving Culture Change

- Determine the culture changes needed and desired based on the current culture of your department.

- Drive successful culture change through broad engagement of your faculty, staff, trainees, and students.
- Be transparent in the rationale, goals, and ongoing metrics for culture change.
- Get help from experts in the field and your institutional HR department.

Promoting Teamwork

- Understand that teamwork reflects constructive cultural attributes of communication, collaboration, and collegiality.
- Promote teamwork among faculty, staff, trainees, and students in order to enhance productivity and innovation in each mission area.
- Communicate and show how teamwork can benefit individual and programmatic success.
- Provide educational programs and practical exercises to demonstrate the benefits of teamwork.
- Use analogies as appropriate to help explain the function and benefits of good teamwork.
- Be a role model as your department's team leader and an institutional team player.

Chapter 7: Diversity, Equity, and Inclusion

Highlighting the Importance of Diversity, Equity, and Inclusion (DEI)

- Communicate that DEI is a key driver of excellence and enhances all department missions.
- Articulate the harmful historical legacy and current damage resulting from inequities.
- Enforce all policies on harassment, discrimination, and bias.
- Adopt DEI in clinical care to promote health equity and reduce disparities.
- Adopt DEI in education to provide learners with skills to work in diverse communities.
- Adopt DEI in research to improve applicability of findings to all groups.
- Adopt DEI in community engagement to build trust.

DEI Education and Training

- Utilize the wide range of available teaching tools, especially those that utilize active learning.
- Become familiar with publications about DEI and use them in your DEI training programs.

Enhancing and Promoting DEI

- Demonstrate the importance of DEI by considering appointment of a DEI leader in your department who reports to you directly.
- Emphasize that DEI is everyone's responsibility.
- Use best practices in DEI for recruitments, including diverse search committees who have been educated about unconscious and other forms of bias.
- Ensure an inclusive culture by addressing equity in compensation, resource allocations, responsibilities, and opportunities.
- Actively participate in special occasions that celebrate diverse department members and communities.
- Ensure diverse representation of invited speakers, participants and guests, for your department's events.
- Identify, emphasize, and make available career development opportunities, especially for women and those from underrepresented groups.
- Become aware of and avoid "gender" and "minority" taxes.

Measuring Success

- Develop metrics to monitor your department's progress in DEI, which often are available from your institution's DEI officer or external resources.
- Communicate the results of DEI metrics to all stakeholders.
- Respond to identified problems with specific interventions to address and enhance opportunities for all members of your department.

Chapter 8: Building Collaborations and Collegiality

The Value Added

- Promote collaboration and collegiality within and across all the mission activities in your department to enhance success.
- Appreciate that some department members may be reluctant to collaborate because they fear loss of control or having ideas stolen.
- Stimulate collaboration to create synergies and provide access to more resources through creation of interdisciplinary and interdepartmental centers and institutes.
- Encourage collegiality and collaboration to improve morale, well-being, and productivity.
- Establish social functions to help facilitate collaboration and collegiality.
- Promote interactions across a wide range of disciplines beyond medicine to provide additional clinical, educational, research, and community service opportunities.

Research and Clinical Faculty Relationships

- Stimulate collaboration between research and clinical faculty to benefit them both and the department.
- Schedule recurring seminars that combine research and clinical presentations.
- Encourage research and clinical faculty to collaborate in teaching courses together.
- Assign research and clinical faculty to department and institution-wide committees.
- Plan departmental seminars and symposia at which both research and clinical faculty can present their scholarly work.

Stimulating Collaboration

- Use retreats with research and clinical faculty with their students/trainees to brainstorm possible collaborations.
- Use seed funding to stimulate collaborative research projects between research and clinical faculty with their students/trainees in your department and potentially others.
- Involve both research and clinical faculty with their students/trainees in fundraising efforts.
- Consider incorporating financial or other incentives for collaboration into your faculty compensation plan.

Promoting Collegiality

- Promote collegiality to enhance negotiation, teamwork, fundraising, and individual wellness.
- Consider using collegiality as a criterion for promotion and as a component of bonus compensation and awards.
- Be a personal example and role model for collaboration and collegiality.

Chapter 9: Promoting Work-Life Balance

Developing a Successful Departmental Work-Life Balance

- Communicate clearly and frequently to your department that work-life balance impacts well-being and mitigates stress and burnout by enhancing resilience, satisfaction, and performance.
- Explain why work-life balance is important and valued by you and your department.
- Provide advice and be a role model for time management and work-life balance.

Work Time

- Offer flexible work times and remote options as appropriate.
- Recommend that faculty take direct control of their calendars and scheduling.
- Educate department members on efficient and effective uses of communication tools.
- Advise clinicians to consider utilizing decision support tools, work with mid-level providers at their full scope of training, and consult with schedulers to reduce over- and under-bookings.
- Advise researchers to focus on higher impact grants and papers, and consider the cost-benefit of additional staff and technological support.
- Advise educators to consider using online, virtual, and simulation technologies.
- Remind faculty and staff that if they already are too busy at work, they should only say "yes" to any additional tasks if they say "no" and stop doing something else.

Personal Time

- Clarify that department members should not feel guilty for taking personal time.
- Explain why using personal time helps keep oneself refreshed and can enhance their productivity and creativity.
- Suggest ways of using personal time each day for hobbies, non-work interests, social interactions with family and friends, and relaxation.
- Recommend taking occasional vacations that are long enough to disconnect and become refreshed.
- Encourage scheduling vacations and time off well in advance and try to avoid encroachments from work-related activities.
- Remind department members that time with children, spouses/partners, and elderly parents is precious and can't be recaptured years later.
- Explain how personal time benefits mental and physical health.
- Be a role model for making personal time a priority.

Chapter 10: Negotiation

When to Negotiate

Consider negotiating when offered a proposal or counter-proposal if:

- Terms are not acceptable.
- Terms are not explicit.
- There are incorrect assumptions.

- Additional considerations could make a better agreement.
- Greater total value for both parties could be created.

Consider starting a new negotiation in response to a proposal if you are not familiar with the other party or what they might value, or if additional parties may become involved.

How to Negotiate

- Ensure that quantitative, accurate data are used.
- Agree on the anticipated benefits to all parties.
- Dry-run proposals, counter-proposals, and options.
- Avoid confrontation and demands.
- Assess the objective of net benefits to your department.
- Consider consequences of missed opportunities.
- Include trusted intermediaries when they may be helpful.

Do's and Don'ts

- Understand the other positions in the negotiation.
- Base your negotiation on mutual trust and transparency.
- Get advice and assistance as needed.
- Bring in a trusted third party as needed.
- Be careful negotiating with non-trusted parties.
- Document everything, especially final agreements.
- Remember that negotiation is a collaborative process that can identify and secure greater value for all parties.

Chapter 11: Organizing the Department

Leadership Positions

- Create a diverse leadership team with trusted people smarter than you in their areas of expertise.
- Appoint leaders who are committed to the department and able to succeed in a rapidly changing future environment.
- Identify a highly trusted, well-connected faculty or staff member to be your "chief of staff" to provide an informal means of two-way communication with members of the department.

- Cautiously remove problem lieutenants sooner rather than later, and watch your back.
- Carefully determine positions to keep, change, and create with broad input from stakeholders.
- Use leadership positions to kill "sacred cows" and to create "disciples."

Building Your Team

- Create a small "Executive Committee" with your best leaders and team players that meets regularly to track departmental progress and consider all major issues and opportunities.
- Align authority of your team leaders with their responsibility and accountability.
- Provide advice, especially when asked, but don't micromanage faculty and staff leaders and members of their teams.

Divisions and Sections

- Review other departmental models to consider what might work best for yours.
- Examine how your department's structure can greatly facilitate or impede engagement and satisfaction of personnel and overall performance.
- Investigate different ways to structure your department based on missions, services, academic units, programs, and operations.
- Consider using leadership positions (e.g., vice chairs, deputy directors, chiefs) to oversee mission areas and other important activities and programs.

Operations and Administration

- Consider your department's size, complexity, and the relationship of parent organizations as key factors in determining how to organize your administrative structure and operational processes.
- Consolidate and coordinate similar administrative/operational functions across divisions and services wherever possible.
- Consider partnering with other departments to improve administrative and operational performance, better utilize resources, and stimulate collaboration.
- Negotiate and develop mutually agreeable approaches to manage personnel, operations, or budgets that are controlled by parent organizations.

Meetings and Events

- Plan to attend your "Executive Committee," "Faculty," and other department-wide meetings as often as possible.

- Be engaging and humble at meetings and events rather than domineering and intimidating.
- Provide education for faculty and staff on how to hold effective meetings.
- Recommend that all departmental meetings include an agenda that is shared beforehand.

Chapter 12: Strategic Planning

Evaluating Your Departmental Strategic Plan

- Evaluate the current strategic plan for stakeholder support, meeting expectations, adequacy of assumptions, available resources, and changes in culture or environment.
- Document any problems and share them with your faculty and institutional leadership.
- Determine whether to utilize or modify/refresh the existing plan, or develop a new plan.

Refreshing an Existing Strategic Plan

- Consider modifying/refreshing the current plan if it was recently developed and now inadequate, and there is resistance or insufficient resources for a new plan.
- Spend minimal time and resources, and address major expectations and priorities when modifying/refreshing an existing plan.

Developing a New Strategic Plan

- Develop a new strategic plan when the current plan is old (>5 years), inadequate, or if there is a clear expectation by institutional leadership that a new plan is needed.
- Assess the level of faculty/staff support and available resources for developing a new plan.
- Take ownership and actively lead the strategic planning process.
- Engage stakeholders in articulating your department's mission and values, agreeing on a vision of achievements with a set timeline, and taking ownership of the results.
- Identify a few key strategic priorities (usually less than 5), and the appropriate resources and tactics to achieve them.
- Make sure that your department's goals are put into the context of the strategic priorities.

- Ensure that strategic plan priorities and their timing are appropriate to your mission, vision, and values, and are realistic for your environment and potential resources.
- Use the priorities of the plan to drive resource allocation and budget processes.
- Consider using a professional facilitator or consultant in helping to develop your plan.
- Assign a leader to each strategic priority with the appropriate responsibility and authority to advance their component of the plan.

Managing Change

- Understand and communicate to your department and institution that the vision, goals, and expectations of your strategic plan will require changes.
- Tailor your change management process to the reasons, expectations, time frame, anticipated resistance, and capacity of you and your team to lead it.
- Utilize the extensive literature as well as advice, coaching, and consultants as needed to manage change.

Chapter 13: Resources

Resource Management

- Appreciate that people are your most important and usually most expensive resource.
- Understand that priorities of your strategic plan are directly linked to the faculty and staff needed for implementation.
- Prioritize resources to be in alignment with your strategic plan and tactics.
- Prioritize programs by evaluating their cost-benefit in consideration of the sources and uses of the resources they need.

People

- Ensure that recruitment and retention of faculty and staff support programmatic strategic priorities.
- Consider the potential advantages and disadvantages of recruiting faculty jointly with other departments and centers.
- Prioritize staff support to assist faculty who have the greatest potential for increased productivity and generation of additional resources.
- Consider creation of core staffing units to increase productivity and enhance collaboration.

Space

- Appreciate that space is a precious resource with limited availability.
- Ensure that adequate facilities are available before recruiting personnel or soliciting funds and equipment for a new or expanded program.
- Understand and explain to your faculty and staff the institutional metrics and policies for space assignment.
- Remove space carefully from under-performing faculty based objectively on their productivity, and your department's strategic priorities, goals, and potential reassignment opportunities.
- Be prepared for push-back from faculty when reassigning their space or asking them to move to new space.
- Balance positive and negative aspects of relocating faculty and programs with appropriate incentives as needed.

Funding

- Make sure you and appropriate department leaders understand institutional funds flows.
- Meet regularly with department and institution financial officers for status reports.
- Determine what expenses are appropriate to fund from operating budget, reserves, and start-up package.
- Examine departmental income sources for missed opportunities as well as hidden deficits and obligations.
- Review long-term financial commitments and their need for continuation.
- Keep your budget balanced and maintain only a modest reserve.

Chapter 14: Budgets and Finance

Assessing Departmental Finances

- Understand your department's profit and losses, assets and liabilities, and cash flow.
- Demonstrate an interest in the financial health and fiscal policies of your institution(s).

Sources and Uses

- Prioritize expenses in your budget process for your department's strategic priorities, goals, and expectations.

- Scrutinize overhead expenses and compare them to internal and external benchmarks.
- Evaluate any cross-subsidies within and between departments, and explain them to your faculty and staff to help address controversy and reduce conflict.
- Challenge high-priority programs to identify additional activities that generate net revenue, especially philanthropy.
- Consider adjusting expenses (while closely monitoring for unintended adverse consequences) to help your financial status by:

    - Using contract staff and consultants rather than full-time employees.
    - Employing part-time faculty or fellows rather than full-time faculty.
    - Utilizing non-tenure clinical, research, or teaching tracks when appropriate.
    - Buying-out full-time tenured faculty who are unproductive.
    - Comparing rental versus purchase of space.
    - Evaluating lease versus purchase options for equipment.

Developing a Budget

- Ensure that your budget process is closely tied to the priorities of your strategic plan.
- Determine if your budget process should be incremental (built on an existing budget), zero-based (starting from scratch), or a combination for different segments of your department.
- Evaluate the accuracy of your revenue and expense assumptions carefully and the factors used in their assessment.
- Consider using outside expert advisors or consultants to improve the stringency of your income and expense assumptions.

Margins and Deficits

- Understand institutional policies and practices for handling anticipated margins and deficits before finalizing your budget.
- Calculate the anticipated impact of any budgeted margins or deficits on the financial health and strategic priorities of your department.
- Alert institutional leaders, your department, and key stakeholders as soon as unanticipated margins or deficits are projected.
- Determine the basis of inaccurate budget assumptions for any unexpected deficits and margins.
- Engage institutional leadership in dealing with significant budget variances.
- Remember that institution leaders consider department funds, including margins and deficits, as their own, analogous to how you view funds in your department, so act accordingly.

Chapter 15: Balancing the Missions

The Balancing Act

- Recognize that few faculty can excel in all four missions (education, clinical, research, and public service) and that most will focus on one or two mission areas.
- Try to balance your departmental programs so that they can succeed in all missions.
- Recruit faculty to the appropriate academic track in which they can flourish and receive proper mentorship.
- Ensure that all faculty are engaged in teaching and providing service to the university and community.
- Establish overall departmental and individual faculty goals in each mission area.
- Use agreed-upon metrics to evaluate faculty in each mission area and have faculty maintain documentation of their activities.

Your Involvement in Each Mission

- Demonstrate interest in each mission area and strive to have significant personal activity as appropriate to maintain credibility with your faculty and peers.
- Appreciate that your involvement in mission activities can provide additional options when transitioning from your leadership position.

Alignment of Missions

- Recognize and communicate that mission alignment has a substantial impact on the productivity and potential opportunities for faculty and the department overall.
- Clarify the nature, extent, and rationale for cross-subsidies between clinical, research, educational, and public service activities in your department, AHC/AMC, and institution(s).
- Appreciate that revenues from clinical service and gifts from grateful patients often subsidize other mission areas, potentially causing tension among clinical and nonclinical faculty.
- Address and discuss concerns about cross-subsidies by engaging faculty directly and openly.
- Develop a departmental policy to provide protected time in appropriate circumstances to clinical faculty to extend their academic activities.
- Provide suitable academic expectations for clinical faculty based on their background and career interests.
- Make certain that your budget process and annual budget leverage resource allocation across missions and programs to support the strategic priorities and tactics.

- Ensure that clinical activity of faculty members informs their teaching and scholarly activities to enhance their productivity across missions.
- Identify and develop areas of synergy across missions for individual faculty as well as for departmental programs.

Chapter 16: Crisis Management

General

- Recognize that crises are time-sensitive, pose significant risks, and require difficult decisions.
- Deal with crises calmly, objectively, and urgently; give them precedence over normal activities; be a role model for others.
- Know the crisis and risk management teams at your institution(s) and how they operate.
- Appoint a crisis management team from your departmental leadership.
- Appreciate that a crisis is often compound, involving several inter-related crises, as well as complex, requiring extensive assessment of problems and potential solutions.
- Evaluate the causes and potential consequences of a crisis to determine possible solutions.
- Get advice from institutional leaders, peers, and outside experts.
- Understand that effective communication with your department and institution is essential when dealing with a crisis.

Financial

- Study trends and review assumptions to anticipate when a financial crisis might occur and develop appropriate contingency plans.
- Determine whether they are due to revenue shortfall, increased expenses, or both.
- Establish whether they are likely to be a one-time or ongoing problem.
- Discuss potential solutions with institutional leadership before implementation.

Environmental

- Understand that environmental crises usually impact the entire institution and region, which may require your attention beyond focusing on the impact on your department.
- Be prepared to work with your institution, government agencies, and service organizations.
- Keep leadership informed of progress and problems in resolving issues.
- Prioritize staffing levels and consider appropriate rationing of services.

Personal

- Evaluate your level of distraction and reduced time commitment for your department.
- Delegate more authority as appropriate and consider if a leave of absence is best.

Opportunities to Learn from Crises

- Understand the importance of effective communication, leadership, teamwork, resilience, rapid planning and implementation, and flexibility.
- Seize opportunities to create transformational changes that would not be otherwise possible.

Chapter 17: Faculty Recruitment and Retention

Recruiting New Faculty

- Consider the rationale for creating new faculty positions and confirm that resources are available for their ongoing support.
- Examine open positions for their flexibility, why they are vacant, and how are they budgeted.
- Use best practices for recruiting diverse candidates that includes awareness about unconscious and other forms of bias.
- Consider the potential value of using a search firm to increase the candidate pool and help in the process.
- Ensure that candidates are a good fit professionally and culturally.
- Determine why a candidate is available and their motivation for moving.
- Consider the relative benefits of junior versus senior candidates and internal versus external candidates based on the specific position and situation.
- Calculate the appropriate start-up package using standardized approaches based on roles, responsibilities, seniority, and stature of the recruited faculty member.
- Be aware of institutional policies and criteria regarding what can and cannot be offered to recruits, especially concerning perks and expenditure of their recruitment funds.
- Develop an effective onboarding process to provide a smooth transition for new faculty.

Retaining Current Talent

- Evaluate the relative benefits and net expense in time and resources for a retention versus a recruitment to fill the position.

- Be on the alert for game-playing and don't get into bidding wars.
- Be supportive of a faculty member leaving if it is in their best career and personal interests.

Closing the Deal

- Consider resource needs for the candidate to be successful and allowable perks such as signing bonuses, parking, tuition recovery, and reimbursed memberships.
- Consider personal needs of the candidate such as mentors, education expenses, family issues, housing, protected time, and career guidance.
- Consider reverse site visits to final candidates.
- Carefully weigh the cost and benefits of expending extra resources to recruit or retain "superstars."
- Avoid waiving policies and standards to recruit or retain anyone.
- Avoid contentious negotiation and consider using an intermediary if a conflict arises.

Appointments, Promotions, and Tenure

- Make sure that you and your faculty understand the APT processes for different tracks and ranks at your institution.
- Handle any disagreements with your departmental APT committee's recommendations carefully with a clear explanation to the committee, the candidate, and the institution.
- Understand the differences between faculty physicians and employed (non-faculty) staff physicians, including roles in departmental votes and planning and differences in compensation.
- Be familiar with policies about emeriti faculty.
- Ensure that hospital credentialing policies are followed for all clinicians, including faculty physicians, staff physicians, and emeriti faculty with clinical privileges.

Chapter 18: Faculty Career Development and Wellness

Resources for Career Development

- Evaluate and provide information to faculty about career development and mentoring programs offered by your institution and professional societies.

- Assist and advise faculty who are interested in enhancing their leadership and management skills about appropriate executive education and business school courses.

Implementing Career Development Programs

- Provide all new and junior faculty with mentors/advisors to help them in their professional activities and career advancement.
- Consider appointing a departmental leader to oversee faculty affairs, including career development, wellness, and mentoring programs.

Expanding Faculty Productivity

- Develop and implement incentives for increasing faculty clinical, education, and research achievements.
- Establish and monitor faculty productivity measures carefully.
- Provide personal advice and contacts to help expand faculty collaborations and productivity, especially across disciplines.

Enhancing Wellness

- Emphasize the importance to faculty of work-life balance, resilience, and personal satisfaction.
- Identify and provide faculty with information about effective approaches for enhancing wellness and mitigating burnout.
- Incorporate efficient time management strategies and reduce workload through redesign whenever possible.
- Create strong support systems to help faculty define and achieve their personal goals.
- Engage faculty and staff in departmental planning and decision-making.

Reviewing Performance

- Be sure that your faculty review processes are clearly defined, consistent with institutional procedures, and well-understood by faculty.
- Ensure that all faculty receive a performance review relative to expectations at least annually.
- Include a discussion of plans and expectation for the coming year, career development, work-life balance and well-being, and potential problems and opportunities during faculty reviews.

- Avoid conflicts of interest and involve objective surrogates in reviews of faculty close to you professionally or personally.

Chapter 19: Faculty Compensation Plans

Characteristics

- Consider multiple components in your compensation plan including base salary, market adjustment for roles and responsibilities, incentive bonus, benefits, discretionary funds, and nonfinancial rewards.
- Examine regional and national salary benchmarks.
- Determine the level of department faculty satisfaction with your compensation plan.
- Engage faculty in developing and modifying the plan.
- Review the plan annually.
- Ensure the plan is equitable and transparent to all faculty.

Incentives and Bonuses

- Consider establishing an incentive bonus plan to help stimulate and reward faculty achievements.
- Determine if individual incentives should be dependent on the achievement of departmental and institutional goals.
- Consider incentives for research excellence that might include exceptional grant support, publications, citations, invited talks, and awards.
- Consider incentives for clinical service excellence that might include patient satisfaction, quality outcomes, length of stay, RVU generation, patient/case workload, and service awards.
- Consider incentives for education excellence that might include exceptional educational grant support, publications, citations, invited talks, and awards.
- Consider incentives for public service excellence that might include exceptional citations, mentorship/sponsorship, and local, regional, and national leadership positions.
- Establish quantitative metrics for each parameter used for incentive bonuses.
- Ensure that your faculty incentive plan is consistent with institutional policies.

Review Process

- Evaluate the productivity of each faculty member at least annually based on explicit expectations made during their prior review.
- Carefully evaluate and discuss requests by faculty to reduce clinical time to pursue more academic activities for the potential impact on their compensation.

- Consider developing a bridge funding program for productive faculty who lose grants as part of your budget and strategic planning processes.
- Include clear guidelines for dealing with nonproductive faculty in your compensation plan.
- Determine the reasons why a faculty member may be unproductive and address potential solutions with them carefully.
- Confirm institutional policies and engage institutional leaders before initiating a faculty reassignment, salary reduction, or dismissal process.

Chapter 20: Dealing with Difficult Faculty

Considerations

- Help faculty to be as productive and successful as possible and fully develop their academic potential.
- Deal quickly and firmly with faculty whose conduct creates problems, which can include inappropriate or improper behavior, violations of policies, refusal to follow expectations, inappropriate use of resources, and illegal activity.
- Identify factors such as tenure status, underrepresented group status, departmental position, prior issues, health status, and nature of a complaint (formal versus informal).

Evaluation

- Use objective and transparent expectations of professional activity and conduct for evaluating transgressions.
- Determine specifics of the situation and document all relevant information.
- Try to understand the perspective of the faculty member.
- Document all interactions and be transparent.
- Engage appropriate departmental and institutional leaders, HR, and legal counsel as needed.
- Follow institutional guidelines and legal regulations.
- Consider use of an objective third party, ombudsperson, and consultant in the evaluation.

Resolution

- Address issues directly, dispassionately, and objectively.
- Develop a range of remedial steps for resolution and negotiate possible alternatives and appropriate compromises.
- Engage at least one other departmental or institutional leader in the resolution process.

Mistakes

- Trying to be unduly considerate, not taking an issue seriously enough, and delaying action can each be deleterious to how you are perceived as a leader, and the culture of your department.
- Not following established protocols and policies, not having sufficient documentation, and not getting advice and institutional approval before offering solutions can each prevent resolution and create significant liability problems for you and the institution.

Chapter 21: Student and Trainee Recruitment

Attracting the Right Students and Trainees

- Prioritize education and emphasize respect for students and trainees.
- Invest in students and trainees—they may be your future recruits and colleagues.
- Highlight electives with open houses and create special interest groups (SIGs).
- Create opportunities for students and trainees to meet and interact with faculty who share their life experience.
- Explore multidisciplinary educational opportunities with other departments and centers.
- Assess programs to provide rotations for medical students from other institutions to highlight your department nationally and identify potential future residents.
- Organize resident and fellow recruitment visits carefully, review recruitment materials, personalize itineraries, and provide warm welcoming comments.
- Appreciate that Master's and PhD students and postdoctoral scholars are key contributors to the academic environment in your department.
- Ensure that you and your faculty interact with your institution's graduate training programs.
- Encourage your faculty to participate on research and clinical training grants.

Providing a High-Quality Learning Environment

- Provide faculty with student evaluations and feedback to continuously help improve the curriculum.
- Incorporate evolving pedagogy and new technology into the student curriculum and trainee experience.
- Interact closely with school GME leaders to optimize resident training.
- Promote diversity, equity, and inclusion with holistic admissions.
- Examine your education programs for inclusion of diverse patients, communities, and medical issues.
- Address student and trainee complaints quickly, and engage HR, deans, DIO, and other experts as appropriate.

- Ensure a timely, fair, and equitable evaluation process for all trainees.
- Take student and trainee complaints seriously and partner with leaders to investigate and address concerns.
- Ensure that training programs are focused on education rather than as an inexpensive or alternative way to provide service.

Providing Compensation and Benefits

- Understand and oversee trainee compensation and benefits to ensure they are equitable and competitive.
- Regularly review regional and national benchmarks of trainee compensation and benefits.
- Stay informed about emerging issues, such as unionization of fellows and post-doctoral scholars.

Chapter 22: Student and Trainee Career Development and Wellness

Resources for Career Development

- Provide career development offerings as an investment in the next generation and potentially in future faculty recruits.
- Ensure availability of mentors from academia and beyond, such as industry and government.
- Consider providing access to training in leadership, time management, negotiation, and other skills.
- Shape departmental culture to provide "personal touches" that can guide students and trainees.

Enhancing Achievement

- Determine the nature and amount of teaching and training that you personally will do as chair.
- Create an inclusive, support environment that is free of harassment and bias.
- Periodically review student and trainee assessments of your department; don't wait for complaints or an accreditation review.
- Provide faculty training and skill assessment in new pedagogical approaches and education technology.
- Consider how to reward expert teachers and whether to create a "master educator" academy.

Promoting Wellness

- Be familiar with institutional and national resources for supporting student and trainee wellness.
- Communicate availability of resources to students and trainees during each orientation and review them when issues arise.
- Ensure that student and trainee mental health issues are addressed compassionately and expeditiously.

Reviewing Performance

- Communicate standardized evaluation policies and procedures to all evaluators, as well as students and trainees.
- Ensure timely feedback on performance, with clearly defined opportunities for improvement.
- Conduct periodic reviews to determine trends in student and trainee performance, including use of national benchmarks.
- Address student and trainee performance issues forthrightly; do not just pass the problem on to the next rotation or position.
- Understand which serious problems (e.g., patient errors, research misconduct, etc.) require reporting to institutional and other regulatory officials.

Chapter 23: Dealing with Difficult Students and Trainees

Considerations

- Encourage faculty to provide feedback proactively and address performance issues as part of the educational process.
- Understand institutional policies and know which leaders (student advisors, education deans, DIO, GME program leads) are responsible for addressing student and trainee problems.
- Be familiar with the issues that require external reporting and work closely with institutional leaders and legal counsel in such cases.

Evaluation

- Be familiar with the institutional and national resources available to help deal with students and trainees who are experiencing difficulties.
- Include information to students/trainees in their orientation about wellness resources and where they can ask for assistance.
- Periodically review any trends in the department regarding student or trainee difficulties and address them proactively.

Resolution

- Ensure that poor performance by students and trainees is addressed early and that interventions are assessed to determine improvements.
- Work with education experts and leaders in your department and institution(s) to develop corrective plans for problem students/trainees and monitor progress.
- Get advice from HR, education deans, and others if asked for a reference check about a student or trainee who experienced difficulties during training in your department.

Mistakes

- Distinguish between mistakes that are expected for trainees and serious errors or lapses in judgment or professionalism.
- Engage institutional leaders, national peers, communications staff, and legal counsel to determine best practices in responding to mistakes.
- Ensure that any required reporting to regulatory, accreditation, or legal authorities is made in a timely and thorough manner.

Chapter 24: Staff Recruitment and Retention

Identifying the Right People for the Jobs

- Appreciate that having high-quality staff is key to your success as chair and to the success of the department.
- As a new chair, meet with key existing staff members to determine fit, establish good working relationships, and clarify bidirectional expectations and aspirations.
- Understand both the "formal" official and the "informal" organizational structures in your department.
- Clarify reporting roles, especially for those staff who report to supervisors outside of the department or who have dual reporting.
- Consider whether shared service models or other partnerships could increase efficiency, productivity, and workforce morale in your department.
- Periodically evaluate DEI issues regarding your staff, including equity in compensation and benefits.
- Strive to create an inclusive work environment which recognizes and rewards the contributions of all employees.
- Pay particular attention to critical hires, especially the senior department administrator and your personal executive assistant.

Recruiting New Staff

- When recruiting for a new position, determine if internal candidates are available and if you also should recruit external candidates.
- Develop standardized recruitment policies and practices regarding advertising, interview processes, selection procedures, extending offers, setting compensation, and onboarding.
- Use recruitments as an opportunity to assess and extend diversity of your staff, including search committee education and development of the interview itinerary.

Retaining Current Staff

- Celebrate existing staff with formal recognition events and smaller day-to-day "thank yous."
- Inform institutional leaders about major accomplishments and honors received by staff.
- Establish clear work policies, such as remote or virtual work options, and implement them equitably to balance benefits to the employee and the department as a whole.

Chapter 25: Staff Career Development and Wellness

Career Development, Succession Planning, and Training

- Identify internal and external training opportunities that can be made available to staff who wish to develop further in their career.
- Consider the development of "career ladders" for employees to help staff attain their full potential and to enhance their retention.
- Provide opportunities for staff to be assigned mentors and to serve as them for others.
- Develop succession plans for key staff positions to ensure smooth operations during staff transitions.
- Identify current staff as "ready now," "ready in 1–2 years," or "ready in 3–5 years" to facilitate staff transitions and plan job promotions appropriately.

Enhancing Productivity

- Incentivize high performance through staff recognition programs for both individuals and teams.

- Use recognition programs to augment compensation, but not as substitutes for competitive and equitable salary and benefits.
- Participate in staff meetings to provide updates, enhance collegiality and teamwork, and thank and congratulate staff for their contributions.

Promoting Wellness

- Identify and communicate the availability of wellness programs to all staff, both during their onboarding and periodically at staff meetings.
- Involve appropriate staff members in key hiring, strategic planning, and operational decisions to ensure authentic engagement in the department.

Reviewing Performance

- Utilize formal performance reviews as an opportunity for formative as well as summative feedback to staff employees.
- Ensure that policies and procedures for performance evaluations are transparent and equitable.
- Ensure that each staff member is provided documentation of their supervisor's annual assessment and agreed upon goals for the upcoming year.
- Provide ongoing, continuous feedback (both positive and constructive negative reviews) in order to help staff optimize their performance.
- Document all corrective action plans and use them to guide interventions, especially for negative reviews if improvement is not sufficient.

Chapter 26 Highlights: Staff Compensation

Salaries and Benefits

- Understand institutional and departmental policies and practices for how salaries and benefits are set for your staff.
- Become familiar with the provisions of any union contracts, including those for administrative staff, house staff, postdoctoral scholars, faculty, and staff physicians.
- Address tensions that may arise when unionized and non-unionized staff work "side-by-side."
- Ensure salary equity with periodic reviews to detect bias and check for internal consistency.

Work Assignments

- Ensure equitable distribution of workload among staff.
- Avoid occupational segregation and stereotyping on the basis of gender, race/ethnicity, and other characteristics.
- Recognize and avoid "minority" taxes, "loyalty taxes," and other forms of inequity in salary and benefits.
- Ensure that compensation is adjusted relative to changes in work assignments.
- Work closely with institutional leaders if staff go on strike to implement contingency plans and maintain essential services, to support the institution in reaching a fair settlement, and in ensuring a smooth return to work after the strike is resolved.

Monitoring Staff Compensation Levels and Equity

- Periodically review salaries and benefits of your staff.
- Develop a close working relationship with HR.
- Use institutional, regional, and national benchmarks to improve competitiveness of compensation in your department.
- Determine the direct and indirect financial impact on revenue and expenses of losing staff because of below-market compensation in comparison to raising compensation to competitive levels.
- If applicable, proactively address relationships of staff (non-faculty) and faculty physicians in the department and in your affiliated hospital.

Chapter 27: Dealing with Difficult or Unproductive Staff

Considerations

- Be a role model for other supervisors by providing proactive feedback to your direct staff reports.
- Set expectations and provide training for supervisors to deal forthrightly with challenging staff issues.
- Don't allow staff to bypass their supervisors to come to you with complaints, unless it involves their supervisor.
- Ensure that all staff understand complaint processes and the availability of resources to help them if they have difficulty with their job or personal responsibilities.

Evaluation and Resolution

- Establish equitable and transparent written standards of conduct and job performance expectations for all your departmental staff.

- Ensure that your departmental standards and expectations align with those of the institution and across all worksites.
- Carefully assess the underlying reasons for staff problems and poor performance, including difficulties at home, medical issues, inadequate training, and inappropriate job fit.
- Utilize internal and external resources to support staff who are experiencing challenges, such as training programs, coaches, employee counseling, and emergency assistance.
- Address problems with staff promptly.
- Do not allow poor staff performance to impact departmental operations.
- Periodically assess departmental trends in staff performance and problems, including reviewing staff satisfaction surveys.

Mistakes

- Address staff mistakes quickly and forthrightly and develop written corrective action plans in conjunction with HR experts, legal counsel, and other institutional leaders as appropriate.
- Carefully document mistakes and poor performance, which will be critical if difficult decisions, including termination, need to be considered.
- Consult HR, legal, and other experts before responding to reference requests for employees who experienced difficulties or left the department under adverse circumstances.

Chapter 28: Interacting with Institutional Leaders

Understanding Your Institutional Leadership Teams

- Understand your institution leadership structure, relationships, priorities, operating model, governance, and culture.
- Determine with whom to interact for different issues and opportunities, as well as how to engage them effectively.
- Know to whom your boss (or bosses) report, what teams they are on, and what teams they lead.
- Understand the authority and responsibility of your peer leaders.

Working with Your Institutional Leaders

- Never go to your boss(es) around or behind their back, especially in a disagreement.
- Meet to share good news, updates, and achievements, not just problems and requests.

- Interact with their staff when possible and as appropriate.
- Behave with them as you would want your own unit leaders to behave with you.

  Dealing with more than one boss (e.g., a dean and hospital director):

- Demonstrate engagement and commitment to the success of their institutions.
- Avoid taking sides when there is tension or disagreement between them.
- Be transparent with both if you are asked for a position on a contentious issue.
- Do not make requests that will benefit one at the expense of another.
- Promote alignment between their organizations.

  Bringing problems or opportunities:

- Never bring a problem without potential solutions.
- Avoid bringing departmental conflicts; it's your job not theirs.
- Be objective and dispassionate in a conflict; try to understand their point of view and that they have other priorities and limited resources.
- Detail the institutional benefits for a departmental request or solution to a problem.
- Avoid giving them surprises and provide a heads-up when a serious problem is looming.
- Be judicious and limit the number of problems or issues brought forward.

Being a Team Player

- Remember you are part of the institutional leadership team and act accordingly in leading your department.
- Always represent the interests of the institutions as well as your department and strive to project an institutional as well as departmental image.
- Be a constructive problem solver to try to improve your AHC/AMC as well as your department.
- Align the interests and priorities of your department with those of your AHC/AMC, the way you would want your faculty to place the interests and priorities of their programs and units with those of the department.

Chapter 29: Interdepartmental Interactions

Working with Peer Institutional Leaders

- Recognize that there are many types of relationships with peers including social, "one-offs," long-term/strategic affiliations, and true partnerships built on trust and mutual support.
- Understand that interdepartmental interactions are influenced by behavior of their leaders, alignment of recognitions/rewards, and organizational structure.

Developing Joint Programs

- Appreciate the research, education, patient care, and public service missions of other departments/centers and how they overlap and differ from your department.
- Try to develop collaborative programs with other departments/centers to create synergies, recruit new talented faculty with joint appointments, and diminish competition.
- Consider scheduling joint conferences, seminars, and meetings to discuss areas of mutual interest in order to facilitate partnerships.
- Explore potential new interdisciplinary clinical product lines, educational offerings, and research programs with other departments and centers.

Resources and Recognition

- Articulate your department's mission and achievements to help peer leaders understand and consider what collaborative opportunities might be of mutual benefit.
- Identify ways that your department can work together with other units to reduce costs through operational efficiencies and shared services.
- Ensure that joint programs provide a net benefit for each participant contributing resources.

Dealing with Interdepartmental Conflicts

- Realize that conflicts most often involve financial, programmatic, personnel, or operational issues.
- Try to initially resolve conflicts informally and face to face.
- Document unsuccessful resolution of conflicts in writing and escalate to the appropriate institutional leader.
- Use professional conflict-resolution experts to assist in difficult cases.
- Understand that conflicts are often prolonged or unresolved with weak or disinterested institutional leaders.
- Avoid allowing departmental conflicts to harm your personal relationships with peers and those to whom you report.

Chapter 30: Departmental and Institutional Alignment

Determining Priorities

- Be sure that you, your faculty, and your staff understand and embrace the institutional mission, values, and vision.

- Develop departmental priorities to be consistent with institutional mission and vision.
- Embed the priorities of your department and institution(s) within your department's strategic plan.
- Carefully consider how to align with parent institutions that conflict with each other in their mission, vision, values, priorities, or expectations.

Misalignment with Institutional Mission and Vision

- Appreciate that misalignment will inevitably lead to conflict between your department and parent institution(s) regarding strategic priorities.
- Determine the cause of any departmental and institutional misalignment of mission or vision, and modify your department's strategic plan as necessary to rectify.
- Realize that ongoing misalignment with your institution(s) may result in their reducing resources provided, micromanaging you and your department, and your possible dismissal.

Building Alignment

- Consider using professional consultants to develop plans for alignment and to achieve consensus.
- Recognize that institutional alignments can be affected by changes in organizational structure and the replacement of leaders.
- Realize that functional alignment of medical schools and teaching hospitals is more effective than structural integration in achieving alignment and enhanced performance.
- Understand that institutional leaders view department resources as their own, and the department chair as leading a part of their organization.
- Appreciate that the institution may develop better opportunities and higher priorities for use of resources that had been considered for your department.
- Demonstrate teamwork and courage by supporting an institutional viewpoint when it may not seem to be in the best interest of your department.
- Help your faculty and staff understand when the interests and priorities of the institution must outweigh those of the department; if the institution flourishes and you maintain a positive relationship, the department ultimately will benefit.

Chapter 31: Interactions with External Entities

Getting Institutional Approval

- Understand your institutional communication policies and practices for interacting with other organizations, especially concerning conflicts of interest, nondisclosure agreements, and prior relationships.

- Determine before an interaction if it will be worth the potential time and effort needed to develop and execute a program.
- Review the approval process of your institution(s) before any agreement that results from an interaction.

Universities

- Appreciate that other universities may have programs that your AMC doesn't and vice versa.
- Consider research and education opportunities for developing joint programs.
- Develop a trusting relationship with partner university leaders who share values and priorities.
- Determine how adjunct faculty appointments at both institutions can provide value.
- Recognize that partnerships can become problematic when institutional conditions or leaders change.

Hospitals and Health Systems

- Examine how general and specialty (e.g., children's, cancer) regional hospitals might be sites for student/resident education, clinical trials, health services research, and clinical consultation.
- Be careful of potential conflicts (e.g., competition for patients), poaching of faculty, and risks to the brand of your unit and institution.
- Make sure agreements have transparent and mutually agreeable termination clauses.

Professional Societies

- Appreciate that many opportunities exist for interactions of mutual benefit that can provide substantial career development opportunities for faculty/staff.
- Consider the potential risk of faculty/departmental resources subsidizing activities with professional and academic societies.
- Assure appropriate departmental and institutional approvals are obtained, especially for conflicts of interest and commitment, before allowing faculty to collaborate or consult.

Nonprofit Organizations

- Determine institutional policy for indirect cost recovery for grants from foundations and nonprofit organizations, which is usually lower than the rate for government grants.

Companies

- Consider the significant research, clinical care, and educational opportunities that may exist for your faculty, department, and institution.
- Be aware that companies value profits, intellectual property, and nondisclosure, which can be incompatible with your institution's policies.
- Review faculty consulting agreements carefully to avoid potential conflicts.

Community Leaders

- Develop personal relationships with institutional board members that can be beneficial to you and the department.
- Engage community leaders as appropriate to help in recruiting faculty and funding programs.
- Be alert to faculty/staff "end-runs" with community leaders attempting to pressure you or your bosses to act on issues that influence your oversight.

The Media

- Realize that while the media can create broad recognition about you, your faculty, staff, and programs, it can also be inaccurate and misleading.
- Engage your institutional media experts even if the media approaches you directly.
- Educate your faculty/staff about risks of inaccurate representations by media.
- Resist responding if you receive personal attacks from the media—consult your communication/PR office for advice and assistance.

Chapter 32: Fundraising and Donor Development

Identifying Uses

- Target fundraising activities on high priorities for the donor and your department.
- Recognize that discretionary unrestricted funds are the most flexible and desirable.
- Seek endowments to support faculty chairs, student scholarships and fellowships, research programs, awards, named lectureships, departmental programs and initiatives.
- Avoid soliciting gifts for operating and administrative expenses and accepting gifts that cost more to maintain than the amount of the gift itself.

Developing Donors

- Develop a strong, trusting relationship with donors, especially by demonstrating prior donor satisfaction with gifts they have made.
- Appreciate that donors consider their contributions as investments that must be shepherded appropriately.
- Provide potential donors with education about the department and specific areas of their interest.
- Partner with other departments to fund raise for interdisciplinary programs.
- Offer a variety of program options and naming opportunities to meet donor priorities.
- Consider establishing a "Board of Visitors/Advisors" of past and potential donors, ensuring that they do not consider themselves to have management or governance authority.
- Use your institutional development team to help identify potential donors, including grateful patients, community members, and department alumni (previous students, faculty, staff).
- Do not divert donations for other uses or activities without the donor's agreement.
- Be cautious and transparent with donors when reducing department resources for programs they have supported.
- Avoid conflicts with others institutional leaders who engage a donor and try to coordinate activity.

Dealing with Foundations

- Understand the foundation's priorities, processes, and organizational model.
- Identify who on the foundation board and administrative team are the important contacts.
- Determine whether the time and effort for engaging with a foundation are worth the opportunity costs.

Creating a Development Program for Your Department

- Be well aligned with your institutional development office and staff.
- Educate and engage your faculty in development and fundraising activities.
- Assess the level of staff support needed to create a development program relative to the actual and opportunity costs involved.
- Base your time commitment for fundraising and development on the potential gift amount, the donor, and program priority.

Chapter 33: Leadership Attributes

Characteristics of Successful Leaders

- Take the job because they have a mission to accomplish.
- Have proper work-life balance, high self-awareness, are well organized, and expert at time management.
- Lead by example, accept responsibility when things go wrong, and follow the chain of command.
- Seek advice, are team oriented, and work for the success of their faculty, staff, and students.

Evaluation of Leadership Skills

- Solicit formal and informal feedback from your faculty and staff, and express appreciation when it is provided.
- Appreciate and use information from the annual and term reviews of your performance to improve.
- Consider your own sense of success as leader and skills that need improvement.

Developing and Maintaining Self-Awareness

- Get candid feedback from trusted sources about your strengths, weaknesses, and behavior.
- Determine what you know and especially what you do not know.
- Be proactive and sincere rather than embarrassed or hesitant to ask for advice and feedback.

Leadership Training

- Understand how training can help you develop and strengthen your leadership skills and self-awareness.
- Seek leadership training through your institution, other organizations, and coaches.

Dealing with Criticism

- Understand that criticism is inevitable for leaders.
- Be objective and don't over-react to criticism.
- Look for constructive aspects of criticism.
- Acknowledge your mistakes and respond with humility when you make them rather than trying to hide them, give excuses, or blame others.

Handling Conflicts of Interest

- Differentiate real and perceived conflicts of interest and commitment.
- Appreciate that conflicts often cannot be resolved completely but usually can be managed.
- Realize that any situation appearing to benefit yourself personally may be considered a conflict of interest by others.

Maintaining Confidentiality

- Try to be transparent, but do not disclose information given in confidence.
- Assume all information provided to you is confidential unless otherwise indicated.
- Understand that you must disclose confidential information if it represents a violation of law or a regulation that mandates reporting.

Chapter 34: Getting Advice and Assistance

Advisors and Consultants

- Use advisors with experience in dealing with the decisions you are facing to help provide recommendations and new ideas.
- Identify peers you know through professional, institutional, or prior relationships as potential advisors.
- Hire professional consultants as external authorities to assist in getting work done when you and your team do not have the time, expertise, or staff available to effectively deal with an issue.

Mentors

- Establish a strong, personal and long-term relationship with mentors as trusted counselors who will help guide you, especially in your career planning and development.
- Consider past or present teachers, supervisors, senior members of your profession or institution, and a member of the search committee that recruited you as potential mentors.
- Determine if your professional societies have senior members who can be used as mentors.
- Utilize several mentors to provide you with different perspectives and viewpoints.

Coaches

- Engage specific performance coaches to help improve your leadership skills by strengthening your areas of weakness and enhancing your areas of strength.
- Hire leadership coaches to help you develop more constructive behaviors and better engage your faculty and institutional leadership.

Sponsors

- Identify advisors, mentors, and professional colleagues who can sponsor you for awards, prizes, professional societies membership, and other leadership positions.
- Provide your sponsors with information and assistance to make their support easy.
- Express gratitude for your sponsor's help, describe the personal impact it may have, and keep them appraised of outcomes.

Family and Friends

- Appreciate the value of family and friends for their trust, candor, and interest in your personal well-being, and their understanding of your personality and values.
- Involve family and trusted friends when considering personal issues such as career choices, self-awareness, and work-life balance.

Chapter 35: Handling Reviews

Dealing with Personal Reviews

- Plan to provide an update on your and the department's progress over the past year.
- Appreciate that your boss(es) may have to use a surrogate for your review.
- Engage the individual who did your review if there are disagreements before going to their superior or anyone else.
- Realize that you may receive a personal review that is initiated off-cycle to deal with perceived performance or behavioral issues.

Purpose of Department Reviews

- Understand that departmental reviews usually focus on department performance under your leadership at the end of your current term, and involve internal or external reviewers or both.
- Appreciate that reviews are often done if you plan to leave your position so that successor candidates can understand concerns and issues.

Preparing for a Department Review

- Presume that a departmental self-study and an anonymous survey of faculty and staff will be required as an initial part of a comprehensive department review.
- Be prepared to identify and recommend external reviewers, and potential department faculty and staff to be interviewed.
- Plan to develop and submit a summary report of your own evaluation of department performance.
- Expect that a focused review on specific areas may only require gathering a few materials.

Review "Etiquette"

- Be straightforward during your session with the committee about your interest and priorities for the future If you wish to be reappointed as chair.
- Be candid in discussing the reasons if you are stepping down.
- Do not ask committee members about their deliberations during their review process.

Dealing with the Review Report

- Accept the findings and recommendations of the review graciously, considering it as a roadmap to improve the performance of you and your department.
- Obtain appropriate permission to share the full or redacted report with the department for the faculty and staff support needed to implement any recommendations.
- Prepare a written response to address recommendations with input from your leadership team.

Dealing with Program and Institution Reviews

- Ensure full departmental engagement with reviews of institutional activities for accreditations and certifications, such as by the LCME, The Joint Commission, AAALAC, and NCI.

Chapter 36: Achieving Work-Life Balance

Importance of Work-Life Balance

- Control your schedule to enhance work-life balance, resilience, and productivity.
- Schedule unstructured time during your workday for unanticipated problems and emergencies.

- Balance the priorities for your work and personal life appropriately.
- Consider taking a sabbatical leave to refresh your personal life and to enhance or retool your professional skills.

Time Management at Work

- Realize that workload and demands on your time increase dramatically from the day you are appointed chair.
- Appreciate that while virtual meetings can save travel time, they also can make your schedule busier.
- Control your calendar personally and have all scheduling handled by trusted assistant(s) who know your priorities and style.

Handling Appointments

- Target meetings for 30 min or less and build in enough time between meetings to reflect on the meeting, write summary notes and follow-up plans, and prepare for the next one.
- Have all appointments considered pending until you explicitly approved them.
- Require those requesting a meeting to send an agenda ahead of time.

Enhancing Resilience

- Make personal time for leisure, physical activities, cultural events, and social engagements.
- Realize that you cannot be effective without taking care of yourself first.

Time for Family and Friends

- Schedule activities and vacations with family and friends well in advance and avoid encroachments from work-related activities.
- Appreciate that family time, especially with children and elderly parents, is limited and precious.

Personal Time

- Do not feel guilty for taking personal time.
- Understand and communicate as a role model that keeping yourself refreshed enhances your resilience, productivity, and creativity, which benefits you and your department.
- Include time each day for personal interests and social interactions.

Chapter 37: Career Transitioning

Knowing When It's Time

- Appreciate the differences in proactively planning a transition to take another leadership position, step down, or retire versus reacting to an imposed transition due to termination, non-renewal, or personal/family issues.
- Proactively consider transitioning when you are no longer stimulated, have become more a manager than leader, do not feel appreciated, have different values and priorities than your boss, or do not have the resources to achieve your departmental or personal expectations.
- Determine your sense of satisfaction and level of engagement with your institution and its leaders when considering a transition.
- Transition while you still have energy, ideas, and a plan to work on something engaging inside or outside your profession.
- Treat the underlying causes before transitioning from burnout, and consider taking a sabbatical or other leave.

Considering Options

- Take enough time to fully evaluate your post-transition opportunities to ensure your activities will be stimulating and keep you satisfied.
- Consider a wide range of options including returning to the faculty, writing, mentoring, working with professional organizations, taking a new leadership position, and moving to a new career.

Imposed Termination

- Work collegially with your institutional leadership to negotiate the best transition possible.
- Appreciate that termination and non-renewal are delicate situations for both you and your supervisor(s), who should be motivated to make it non-contentious for their reputations as well as yours.

Succession Planning

- Appreciate that planning to leave your leadership position creates a difficult period for you and the department.
- Begin contingency succession planning soon after your appointment as a leader, and update it regularly with the review of your strategic plan.

Coping with Transition

- Realize that, if you step down and remain in the department, your lack of authority and not being in the information and decision-making loops may be difficult to accept.
- Determine how you can be of service to your department and your successor after your transition from chair.
- Prepare a written plan for potential activities when transitioning and discuss it with advisors, family, and friends.

Chapter 38: Changing Positions

Becoming a Candidate

- Determine why you want to become a candidate for another position and be able to explain it clearly and concisely.
- Ask sponsors, mentors, and advisors to help you become a candidate for positions in which you have interest.
- Respond to invitations to consider other positions candidly by indicating your potential interest in the new position and your level of satisfaction in your current position.

Interviews and Visits

- Inform those to whom you report if you are invited for a formal candidate visit after an initial screening interview.
- Do your homework before making a candidate visiting by researching the people you will meet, the administrative hierarchy, and the culture and history of the institution.

Evaluating the Opportunity

- Consider professional and personal advantages and disadvantages of a new position, and especially how well you will fit into the culture of the new institution.
- Be sure the roles and responsibilities offered are aligned with the authority provided.
- Be able to succinctly articulate your interest in the new position and what you can bring to it.

Closing the Deal

- Be careful in negotiations and consider using an intermediary to avoid conflicts.
- Consider not only resources, money, and space but also less tangible factors such as your potential influence, colleagues, and institutional affiliations.

Leaving Gracefully

- Create a timeline for your departure that is acceptable to your current and new institutions, and ask the institutions to help resolve any conflicts with priority given to your new institution.
- Try to clear up any unresolved departmental problems before you leave.
- Strive to leave your position in a positive manner to enhance your reputation, your legacy at your previous institution, and your success in your new role.

Expect Surprises

- Anticipate that some aspects of the position may differ from what you expected because they weren't discussed in enough detail or at all.
- Address significant problems in a new job quickly and consider options, especially when if the culture, values, and fit are not right for you, or recruitment promises are not being honored.

Index

A

Academic freedom, 32–33
Accreditation Council for Continuing Medical Education (ACCME), 234
Accreditation Council for Graduate Medical Education (ACGME), 140
Active communication, 206
Advisor, 223–224, 226, 227
American Hospital Association (AHA), 217
Appointments, promotions and tenure (APT) process, 111–113
Assessing departmental finances, 87–88
Association of American Medical Colleges (AAMC), 217
Assumptions, 57
Audience, 27–29
Authority, 7–8

B

Balancing act, 95–96
Bias, 41–46
Body language, 28–30
Budget process, 88, 89, 91, 92
Building alignment, 190–191
Burnout, 54, 56

C

Career development, 1, 45, 163–164
Career ladders, 163
Career transitions, 245
Carol Emmott Fellowship, 45
Center for Creative Leadership, 217
Chair package, 8
Chair's cycle, 246

Chronicle of Higher Education Strategic Leadership Program for Department Chairs, 217–218
Coaches, 225–226
Collaboration
    facilitating, 97
    interdisciplinary, 49
    research and clinical faculty relationships, 50
    stimulation, 51
    value added, 49–50
Colleague, 21
Collegiality, 49–52
Commitment, 23
Communication
    accommodating institutional priorities and reforms, 33–34
    processes, 11
    skills, 27–30
    transparency and establishing trust, 30–33
Community leader, 199–201
Companies, 198–199
Conflict of interest, 219, 220
Confrontation, 58, 59
Consultant, 223, 224, 226, 227
Continuing medical education (CME) programs, 142
Coping with transition, 248–249
COVID pandemic, 102, 119, 120
Crisis management
    environmental crisis, 100, 101
    financial crisis, 100
    personal crisis, 101
    significant and unexpected crisis, 99
    transformational opportunities, 101, 102

Cross-subsidies, 96
Culture change, 37

D
Deficits, 88, 92
Demand-driven recruitment, 105
Demands, 58, 59
Departmental finances, 87, 88
Departmental mission, 76
Departmental organizational model, 67
Departmental resources, 58
Department reviews, 231, 232
Department's mission activities, 95
Department's organization
    divisions and sections, 67–68
    leadership positions, 63–64
    meetings and events, 69–71
    operations and administration, 68–69
    team building, 64–67
Determining priorities, 189
Detrimental physical and mental effects, 242
Development program, 209
Development staff support, 209
Difficult faculty
    considerations, 131–132
    evaluation, 132
    mistakes, 133
    resolution, 132–133
Difficult staff, 173–174
Difficult students and trainees, deal with
    considerations, 151
    evaluation, 152
    mistakes, 153
    resolution, 152–153
Discrimination, 41–44
Diversity, equity, and inclusion (DEI)
    education and training, 42–43
    enhancing and promoting, 43–46
    measuring success, 46
Donor development, 204–208, 210
Drexel University Executive Leadership in
        Academic Medicine (ELAM)
        Program, 217

E
Educating potential donors, 205
Emeriti faculty, 114–115
Endowed entity, 203
Enhancing productivity, 164–165
Enhancing resilience, 241
Environmental crisis, 100, 101

Executive committee, 64–66, 70, 71
Executive Leadership in Academic Medicine
        (ELAM), 117
Expectations
    "internal" *vs.* "external" recruitment, 18
    interim leader, 16–18
    measuring success, 15–16
    prior leadership experience, 18–19
    surprises, 19
Expenses, 87–92
External candidate, 18, 19, 106
External entities, interaction with
    community leaders, 199–201
    companies, 198–199
    getting institutional approval, 193
    hospitals and health systems, 195–196
    media, 201–202
    non-profit organizations, 198
    professional societies, 196–198
    universities, 194
External training programs, 175

F
Facilitating collaboration, 97
Faculty career development and wellness
    enhancing wellness, 120–121
    expanding faculty productivity, 118–119
    implementation, 118
    resources, 117
    reviewing performance, 121–122
Faculty compensation plans
    characteristics, 125–126
    incentives and bonuses, 126–127
    review process, 127–129
Family, 226–227
Financial crisis, 100
Formal/informal "cost-benefit" analysis, 81
Freedom of Information Act (FOIA), 202
Free speech, 33
Friends, 226–227
Funding low priority programs, 89
Fundraising
    foundations, 208, 209
    identification, 203–204
    time and effort, 210
Funds flow, 85–86

H
Handle criticism, 218–219
Handling appointments, 240–241
Handling conflicts of interest, 219–220

Handling meeting, 240–241
Handling reviews
    dealing with personal reviews, 229–231
    dealing with program and institution
        reviews, 234–235
    department reviews, 231, 232
    review etiquette, 233
    review report, 233–234
Harassment, 41, 44
Harvard Executive Leadership Program
    (HELP), 217
High employee turnover, 175
High-functioning staff, 157–158
Hospital affiliations, 196
Hospitals and health systems, 195–196

I
Implicit Association Test (IAT), 44
Imposed termination, 247
Incentives, 51
Inclusive and equitable department, 44
Indirect costs, 209
Institutional finances, 87–88
Institutional leaders, 179–182
Institutional training programs, 175
Interdepartmental clinical programs, 184
Interdepartmental conflicts, 187
Interdepartmental interactions
    developing joint programs, 184–185
        administrative, 185
        clinical, 184
        education, 185
        interdisciplinary research, 184
        public service, 185
    peer institutional leaders, 183
    resources and recognition, 186–187
Interdisciplinary research, 184
Internal candidate, 18, 106
Issue resolution, 174–175

J
Job agreement, 253–254
Job candidacy, 253
Job interviews, 252
Job options, 246–247
Joint recruitment, 82–83

L
Leadership attributes

characteristics of, 213–215
    developing and maintaining self-
        awareness, 216–217
    evaluation of leadership skills, 216
    handle criticism, 218–219
    handling conflicts of interest, 219–220
    leadership training, 217–218
    maintaining confidentiality, 220
Leadership coaching, 225
Leadership opportunity, 253
Leadership skills, 216
Leadership training, 217–218
Learning environment, 146–147
Leaving gracefully, 254
Long-term leadership service, 246
Low staff satisfaction scores, 175

M
Maintaining confidentiality, 220
Managing change, 77–78
Margins, 87–89, 92
Media, 201–202
Medical school department chairs, 1
    complex leadership, 1
    constituents achievement, 2
    different models, 2
    financial operation, 2
    good work life balance development, 2
    interaction with multiple entities, 1
    learning, academic and clinical culture, 2
Mentors, 225, 227
Metrics, 46
Mission alignment, 96–97
"Mission-based" budget, 89
Mission misalignment, 190
Mistakes, 217

N
Negotiation, 57–59
Non-profit organizations, 198

O
Opportunity-driven recruitment, 105
Organizational chart, 158
Organizational culture
    culture types and styles, 35–36
    driving culture change, 37
    evaluation, 36–37
    promoting teamwork, 38

P
Periodic staff satisfaction surveys, 175
Personal crisis, 101
Personal time, 55–56, 242
Post-doctoral researchers' salaries, 143
Predecessor, 21–23
Proactive transition planning, 245
Professional societies, 196–198
Promoting collegiality, 51–52
Promoting teamwork, 38
Promoting wellness, 165
Promoting work-life balance
    personal time, 55–56
    wellness, 53–55
    work time, 54–55
Public recognition, 160
Public service mission, 185

Q
Quadripartite mission, 95
Quantitative metrics, 127
Quiet quitting, 120

R
Recruitment, 106
    appointing search committees, 107
    internal *vs.* external candidates, 106
    research and clinical faculty, 108
    search firms, 107
    types, 105
Regional and national references, 125
Reputation, 23
Research and clinical faculty relationships, 50
Resilience, 241
Resources
    allocation, 81, 84, 85
    equipment, 81–85
    funding, 85–86
    management, 81
    people, 82–83
    space, 84–85
Responsibility, 7–9
Retention, 106, 110–111
Retired faculty, 114
Revenue, 87–91
Review etiquette, 233
Reviewing performance, 165–166
Review report, 233–234
Right people identification for jobs, 157–158
Roadmaps, 163
Rumors, 32

S
Sabbatical leave, 238
Salary equity, 125–129
"Seed grant" funding program, 51
Self-awareness, 216, 217, 246
Setting goals, 9, 10, 12
Sharing professional and social
        interests, 204
Social functions, 120
Space, 81–85
Sponsor, 226
Staff compensation
    monitoring staff compensation levels
            and equity, 169–170
    salaries and benefits, 167–168
    work assignments, 169
Staff distribution, 209
Staff mistakes, 175
Staff recruitment, 159–160
Staff retention, 160–161
Stimulating collaboration, 51
Strategic planning, 73–77
    managing change, 77–78
    tactics, 77
Strengths, weaknesses, opportunities,
        and threats (SWOT)
        analysis, 12, 77
Student and trainee career development and
        wellness
    enhancing achievement, 146–147
    promoting wellness, 147–148
    resources, 145–146
    reviewing performance, 148–149
Student and trainee recruitment
    high-quality learning
            environment, 137–142
    post-doctoral fellows, 140, 142
    providing compensation and
            benefits, 142–143
    residents, 137, 138, 140, 142
Succession planning, 164, 248
Surprises, 254–255

T
Team player, 181–182
Time management, 239
Transformational opportunities, 101, 102

U
"Unlimited" resources, 11
Unproductive staff, 173–174

V
Vision misalignment, 190
Volunteer faculty, 114–115

W
Work-life balance
enhancing resilience, 241
handling appointments, 240–241
personal time, 242
time management at work, 239
time with family and friends, 241–242
Work time, 54–55